PREVENTING
HEART DISEASE

PREVENTING HEART DISEASE

What Every Woman Should Know

RITA BARON-FAUST

*with the Physicians of the New York University
Medical Center Women's Health Service
and the Division of
Cardiology*

HEARST BOOKS

New York

LIBRARY OF CONGRESS CATALOGING-IN-PUBLICATION DATA
Baron-Faust, Rita.
Preventing heart disease : what every woman should know / Rita
Baron-Faust, with the physicians of the New York University Medical
Center Women's Health Service and the Division of Cardiology.
p.   cm.
Includes bibliographical references and index.
ISBN 0-688-12070-9
1. Heart—Diseases—Popular works. 2. Women—Diseases—
Prevention. 3. Heart—Diseases—Prevention. I. Title.
RC672.B373   1995
616.1'205'082—dc20   94-30549 CIP

Printed in the United States of America

First Edition

1 2 3 4 5 6 7 8 9 10

BOOK DESIGN BY KATY RIEGEL

For Dad and Grandpa,
who would have been proud

Series Introduction

FOR FAR TOO long the concept of women's health has been narrowly focused on reproduction and the reproductive organs. This limited view has caused medicine to virtually ignore the presence of coronary artery disease in women, to underfund research into breast cancer, to fail to recognize the symptoms of AIDS unique to women and to view menopause as akin to a disease rather than as one stage in a woman's life cycle.

Today, medicine is beginning to acknowledge what many of us have known for many years: The fragmentation of women's health care costs lives. Women suffer more days of disability resulting from health problems than men, and the gender gap widens with age. Combating this problem requires a comprehensive, interdisciplinary approach to education, clinical care, prevention and research.

The first steps toward this goal were taken in 1990 with the establishment of the Office of Research on Women's Health and the subsequent funding of $625 million for the Women's Health Initiative. Hundreds of studies and clinical trials in women's health are now under way, new efforts are being made to educate physicians better in this field and centers are being established across the country to provide improved health care for women.

New York University Medical Center has combined all three approaches in the NYU Women's Health Service (WHS). Drawing upon the vast scientific resources of a major medical center, women referred to the WHS can take advantage of the latest technology in screening for breast, ovarian and uterine cancer, cardiovascular disease, osteoporosis and metabolic disorders. In addition, state-of-the-art assisted reproductive in-vitro fertilization technology, preventive services and psychological counseling are available. The service also sponsors free community educational seminars.

Founded in 1992, the WHS is a nonprofit venture dedicated to the study of women's health issues. The service supports biomedical and clinical research by the NYU School of Medicine and NYU Medical Center. We are also engaged in clinical trials in a number of fields.

A series of women's health handbooks, *What Every Woman Should Know About* . . . is an extension of our efforts to merge medical research, patient care and community outreach. These handbooks will provide up-to-date scientific information on the prevention, detection and treatment of the major health problems affecting women today, including cardiovascular disease, breast cancer and depression. Armed with the facts, women can take action to avoid many diseases or take steps to detect and treat problems as early as possible. We recognize that cultural differences have a major impact on health behavior. Each handbook will address the concerns of women of different racial and ethnic backgrounds.

In our efforts to reshape medical care in the twenty-first century, we must become more active and informed participants in our own health care. We hope these books will help women accomplish that goal.

—Robert H. Morris, M.D.
Director, New York University Medical Center
Women's Health Service

Preface

OVER THE PAST three decades, science has made great strides in the battle against cardiovascular disease. As a result, deaths from coronary artery disease have been cut in half and there have been comparable declines in deaths from strokes and hypertension.

Many of the research findings and techniques that have led to these advances were pioneered and applied by physicians at the New York University School of Medicine and NYU Medical Center. NYU's contributions to the field of cardiology include the discovery of the thrombolytic agent streptokinase, the first uses of electrophysiology—measurements of the electrical activity—of the heart, the development of cardiac catheterization and the establishment of one of the first centers for coronary bypass surgery.

Cardiologists at NYU and its associated institutions have also been in the forefront of prevention efforts, playing an instrumental role in the establishment of both the New York Heart Association and the American Heart Association.

The publication of *Preventing Heart Disease: What Every Woman Should Know*, the first comprehensive prevention guide for coronary artery disease solely for women, is a continuation of NYU's efforts to conquer this disease, which remains the number one killer of American women. By providing women with the information they need to protect and improve their cardiovascular health, we hope to make even greater progress against heart disease.

      —Larry A. Chinitz, M.D.
        Assistant Professor of Clinical Medicine
        Director, Cardiac Electrophysiology, NYU Medical Center

Foreword

The Female Heart Is Vulnerable to Coronary Disease

CORONARY HEART DISEASE—the disease that results in angina pectoris (chest pain), myocardial infarction (heart attack), and complicating heart failure and disturbances of heart rhythm—is the major cause of death for women in the United States, responsible for about 250,000 deaths each year. Although women generally develop the clinical evidence of coronary heart disease one to two decades later than their male counterparts, women fare worse than do men once coronary disease becomes evident. As an example, women are more likely than men to die both during the hospitalization for a heart attack and during the year that follows; and women have less favorable outcomes after coronary artery bypass surgery and coronary balloon angioplasty procedures. Equally important is the substantial disability of women known to have coronary disease; about 36 percent of women aged fifty-five to sixty-four years are limited in their activities due to symptoms of heart disease, and this percentage rises to 55 percent for women older than seventy-five years of age. Although women live, on average, six to seven years longer than do men, about four of these years are often years of illness; clearly the challenge is to improve for women the quality of these added years.

Equally clearly, prevention of coronary disease is warranted for women, and the preventive efforts must begin at a young age to avert disease later in life. However, unless women consider coronary heart disease to be part of their illness experience, they are unlikely to heed preventive messages and learn the skills needed to undertake preventive strategies. Further, they are unlikely to respond promptly and appropriately to symptoms of chest pain that may signal a heart attack.

Rita Baron-Faust has compiled a spectacular educational resource, highlighting both the importance of prevention and the means of its implementation. Until recent years, coronary heart disease was viewed as a disease of men, and the woman's task was seen as helping her father, spouse, male siblings, and male children reduce their risk of developing this serious illness. The emphasis in this decade is that the female heart is, indeed, vulnerable to coronary heart disease. In recent years, more women than men have died from coronary disease; it is not that women are becoming sicker but that, with aging of the population, larger numbers of women now live to the elderly ages when clinical evidence of coronary heart disease appears. Heeding the preventive messages in this volume should enable informed women to participate in improving their heart health in specific and the public health of our nation in general.

Read and learn! Become a heart health advocate for yourself and for other women! Live longer and healthier!

—Nanette K. Wenger, M.D.
Professor of Medicine (Cardiology)
Emory University School of Medicine

Acknowledgments

I AM INDEBTED to New York University Medical Center, which generously gave its cooperation from the inception of this project. John Deats, then director of public affairs at NYU Medical Center, lent enthusiastic support to the idea and was instrumental in getting it off the ground. As the project progressed from proposal to page, Mark Danes, director of public affairs, and David Sachs, former director of publications, helped to smooth my path inside the institution, as have Dr. Robert Morris and Dr. Robert Porges.

I am especially indebted to Dr. Anthony Grieco for his continued support, insights and encouragement; to Dr. Arthur C. Fox, who assembled a team of cardiac fellows to guide the writing of the initial manuscript; to Dr. Robin Freedberg, who was instrumental in shaping the first draft; and to Dr. Stephen Siegel and Dr. Mariano Rey, who volunteered for extra duty as peer reviewers of my final draft; and to Dr. Larry Chinitz for writing the Preface. My gratitude also to all the physicians and other experts at NYU who acted as medical advisers and who helped me greatly in ensuring the scientific accuracy of the material. In particular, Dr. Herbert Kayden, Dr. Maret Traber and Dr. Jerome Lowenstein, who were tough critics for the chapters on cholesterol and hypertension.

I am also deeply grateful to the patients of NYU's Cooperative Care Unit, Cardiac Rehabilitation Program, Smokeless Program and Weight

Management Program for Women, as well as the other women who so generously shared their stories with me.

Special thanks go to Dr. Marvin Moser of Yale for reviewing the material on hypertension; Dr. William Castelli of the Framingham Heart Study and Dr. James Cleeman of the National Cholesterol Education Campaign for making themselves available as resources; Dr. Nanette Wenger at Emory University for her invaluable insights over the years; Howard Lewis, Ann Williams, John Weeks, Diane Goetz, Phil Kebak, Carol Floyd and Marilyn Allen at the American Heart Association for all their help; Diane Stryer at the National Heart, Lung and Blood Institute; my editor at Hearst Books, Toni Sciarra, from whom I learned a great deal about editing (and cutting copy); and my agent, Vicky Bijur, for her enthusiasm and support. Thanks also go to my research assistant, Natalie Medine, without whose help I could not have written this book; to my husband, Allen, for not minding (too much) all the late nights and for keeping my computer running; to my son, Alexander, for all his "help" in the office; and to my mother, my best critic, who always reads every word.

Stephen A. Siegel, M.D., F.A.C.C.
Co-Director, Cardiac Stress Lab,
Clinical Assistant Professor of Medicine

Mariano J. Rey, M.D.
Director, Cardiac Rehabilitation Program,
Associate Professor of Medicine,
Director, Cardiac Exercise Laboratory

NYU MEDICAL ADVISERS AND PEER REVIEWERS

Mark A. Adelman, M.D.
Assistant Professor of Surgery,
Division of Vascular Surgery

Esther Chachkes, M.S.W.
Director of Social Work, NYU Medical Center
Adjunct Assistant Professor of Social Work,
NYU School of Social Work

Larry A. Chinitz, M.D.
Assistant Professor of Clinical Medicine (Cardiology)
Director, Cardiac Electrophysiology

Jane Cooper, C.S.W., M.S. Ed.
NYU Cooperative Care Education Center

Laura Ann Demopoulos, M.D.
Cardiology Fellow NYU, 1993

Eileen DiFrisco, R.N., M.A.
Senior Nurse-Educator,
Senior Nurse Clinician

Francesca Gany, M.D.
Director, New York Task Force on Immigrant Health,
NYU-Bellevue Hospital Center

Taya V. Glotzker, M.D.
Cardiology Fellow, 1994

Erminia M. Guarneri, M.D.
Cardiology Fellow, 1994

Leigh Ann Hutchinson, M.D.
Cardiology Fellow, 1994

Adina Kalet, M.D., M.P.H.
Director Training Programs,
Gouverneur Hospital Diagnostic Treatment Center,
NYU Medical School, Department of Medicine

Herbert J. Kayden, M.D.
Professor of Medicine,
Director, Lipid Metabolism Laboratory

Itzhak Kronzon, M.D.
Director, Non-Invasive Cardiology,
Professor of Clinical Medicine

Mack Lipkin, Jr., M.D.
Professor of Medicine,
Director, Division of Primary Care and Internal Medicine,
NYU-Bellevue Hospital Center

Jerome Lowenstein, M.D.
Professor of Medicine

Sydney J. Mehl, M.D.
Clinical Associate Professor of Medicine (Cardiology)

Reed C. Moskowitz, M.D.
Medical Director, Stress Disorders Medical Services,
Clinical Assistant Professor of Psychiatry

Lila E. Nachtigall, M.D.
Associate Professor, Obstetrics and Gynecology
Director, Women's Wellness, NYU Women's Health Service

Valerie Peck, M.D.
Clinical Assistant Professor of Medicine,
Medical Co-Director, Bone Density Unit,
NYU Women's Health Service

Horacio D. Pineda, M.D.
Co-Director, Cardiac Rehabilitation Program,
Rusk Institute for Rehabilitation Medicine
Assistant Clinical Professor of Rehabilitation Medicine

Sabina Primack, M.S.W.
Social Work Supervisor, Cardiac Surgery,
NYU Medical Center/Tisch Hospital

Cecilia Schmidt-Sarosi, M.D.
Professor of Obstetrics and Gynecology,
Director of Reproductive Endocrinology and Infertility,
NYU Women's Health Service

Jennifer Stack, R.D.
Senior Nutritionist,
Cooperative Care Outpatient Education Program,
Director, Weight Management Program for Women

Maret G. Traber, Ph.D.
Research Associate Professor,
Lipid Metabolism Laboratory

The author also wishes to express gratitude to the following individuals who graciously provided information, insight and peer review into the issues concerning women and heart disease during the three years of research and writing this book.

Phyllis August, M.D.
Associate Professor of Medicine and Obstetrics and Gynecology,
Cornell University Medical College, New York

Elizabeth L. Barrett-Connor, M.D.
Professor and Chair,
Department of Family and Preventive Medicine
University of California, San Diego School of Medicine

Herbert Benson, M.D.
Director, Mind-Body Institute,
Chief of Behavioral Medicine,
New England Deaconess Hospital, Boston
Professor of Medicine, Harvard Medical School

Nina A. Bickell, M.D., M.P.H.
Senior Medical Research Scientist,
New York State Department of Health,
Office of Quality Improvement

Steven N. Blair, Ph.D.
Director of Epidemiology,
Institute for Aerobics Research, Dallas

Julie E. Buring, Sc.D.
Principal Investigator, Women's Health Study,
Associate Professor of Ambulatory Care and Prevention,
Harvard Medical School/Brigham and Women's Hospital, Boston

Joseph S. Carey, M.D.
Clinical Associate Professor of Surgery,
UCLA Medical Center

William Castelli, M.D.
Director, Framingham Heart Study,
Framingham, Massachusetts

James I. Cleeman, M.D.
Coordinator, National Cholesterol Education Program,
National Heart, Lung and Blood Institute,
National Institutes of Health, Bethesda, Maryland

John R. Crouse, M.D.
Professor of Medicine, Preventive Cardiology,
Bowman Gray School of Medicine, Winston-Salem, North Carolina

Richard O. Cummins, M.D.
Professor of Medicine,
Associate Director, Emergency Medical Services,
University of Washington Medical Center, Seattle

Margo A. Denke, M.D.
Associate Professor,
Department of Internal Medicine,
Center for Human Nutrition
University of Texas Southwestern Medical Center, Dallas

Katherine Detre, M.D., Dr. P.H., F.A.C.C.
Professor of Epidemiology,
University of Pittsburgh

Keith C. Ferdinand, M.D.,
Association of Black Cardiologists, Miami

Stanton A. Glanz, Ph.D.
Professor of Medicine, Division of Cardiology,
University of California at San Francisco

Mark Greenberg, M.D.
Director, Cardiac Catheterization Lab,
Montefiore Medical Center, Bronx, New York
Associate Professor of Medicine and Radiology,
Albert Einstein College of Medicine

Clarence E. Grim, M.D.
Professor of Medicine in Residence,
Director, Drew UCLA Hypertension Research Center,
Charles R. Drew University of Medicine and Science, Los Angeles

Charles Hennekens, M.D.
Director, Physicians Health Study,
Harvard Medical School/Brigham and Women's Hospital, Boston

Mara Julius, Sc.D.
Psychosocial Epidemiologist,
Department of Epidemiology,
School of Public Health, University of Michigan, Ann Arbor

Marjorie Kagawa-Singer, Ph.D., M.N., R.N.
Associate Researcher, National Research Center
for Asian American Mental Health at UCLA, Los Angeles

Sheryl F. Kelsey, Ph.D.
Associate Professor of Epidemiology,
University of Pittsburgh

B. Waine Kong, Ph.D.
Executive Director, Association of Black Cardiologists
Vice President, Medical Affairs, PCA Health Plans, Miami

Nancy Krieger, Ph.D.
Division of Research,
Kaiser Foundation Research Institute, Oakland, California

David Kritchevsky, Ph.D.
Associate Director, Institute Professor,
Wistar Institute, Philadelphia, Pennsylvania
Wistar Professor of Biochemistry, University of Pennsylvania

John C. LaRosa, M.D.
Dean for Research,
Director, Lipid Research Clinic,
George Washington University Medical Center, Washington, D.C.
Chairman, American Heart Association Cholesterol Task Force

Judith H. LaRosa, R.N., Ph.D.
Deputy Director, Office of Research on Women's Health,
National Institutes of Health

JoAnn E. Manson, M.D.
Co-Director, Women's Health,
Harvard Medical School/Brigham and Women's Hospital, Boston
Principal Investigator, Nurses' Health Study

Karen A. Matthews, Ph.D.
Professor of Psychiatry and Epidemiology,
University of Pittsburgh

Marvin Moser, M.D., F.A.C.P.
Clinical Professor of Medicine (Cardiology),
Yale University School of Medicine, New Haven

Hiltrud S. Mueller, M.D.
Associate Director, Division of Cardiology,
Montefiore Medical Center, Bronx, New York
Professor of Medicine, Albert Einstein College of Medicine

Linda Curtis O'Bannon, M.D.
Editor and Publisher, *Urban Physician's Focus*
Attending Physician, Humana-Michael Reese Hospital, Chicago

Gerald T. O'Connor, Ph.D., D.Sc.
Assistant Professor of Medicine and Community and Family Medicine,
Dartmouth-Hitchcock Medical Center, Hanover, New Hampshire

Jane F. Owens, Ph.D.
Department of Epidemiology,
Cardiovascular Behavioral Medicine Program,
Department of Psychiatry,
University of Pittsburgh

Diana B. Petitti, M.D.
Director, Research and Evaluation,
Southern California Kaiser Permanente Medical Group, Pasadena,
    California

Thomas G. Pickering, M.D.
Associate Director, Cardiovascular and Hypertension Center,
New York Hospital-Cornell Medical Center
Professor of Medicine, Cornell University Medical College

Ileana L. Pina, M.D.
Associate Professor of Medicine/Cardiology,
Director Cardiac Rehabilitation,
Acting Director Heart Failure,
Temple University School of Medicine, Philadelphia

Jean Sealy, Sc.D.
Research Professor of Medicine,
Cornell University Medical College, New York

Jane B. Sherwood, R.N., B.S.N.
Research Nurse Manager, MI Onset Study,
New England Deaconess Hospital, Boston
Institute for Prevention of Cardiovascular Disease

Rodman Starke, M.D.
Senior Vice President, Scientific Affairs,
American Heart Association, Dallas, Texas

Nanette Kass Wenger, M.D.
Professor of Medicine (Cardiology),
Emory University School of Medicine, Atlanta

Redford B. Williams, M.D.
Professor of Psychiatry and Psychology,
Associate Professor of Medicine,
Duke University Medical Center, Durham, North Carolina

Contents

PREVENTING
HEART DISEASE

1

Heart Disease—
Not for Men Only

Heart disease? I never thought about my heart at all until I got sick. It never occurred to me that I might be at risk. No one in my family had ever had a heart attack. For a long time, I denied the possibility that the chest pains I was having were related to my heart. I thought men had heart problems, not women.

Margery, age forty-eight, double-bypass patient

HEART DISEASE IS hardly a male affliction. In fact, more women than men—479,359 women, compared to 446,702 men—die each year in America of diseases of the heart and blood vessels, including stroke. That's more than *any* other single disease, including all forms of cancer and AIDS. Yet a 1994 Gallup survey found that 80 percent of women were unaware that heart disease is the leading cause of death among women; over half of the women surveyed felt cancer was a bigger threat to their lives.

According to the American Heart Association, one in nine women between the ages of forty-five and sixty-four have some form of cardiovascular disease. After age sixty-five, the ratio increases to one out of every three women. By the year 2015, almost half of American women will be forty-five years of age or older—and headed for the postmenopausal cardiac danger zone.

When a woman gets there, her chances of dying of heart disease will be higher than a man's: Cardiovascular diseases now account for 51.6

percent of deaths among women, compared with 48.4 percent of deaths among men.

The mistaken idea that heart disease is not a problem for women has led to lack of emphasis on prevention for women. While men and women share the *same* basic risk factors for heart attacks and strokes, many of those risks pose a greater danger to women.

ARE YOU AT RISK?

A 1994 survey by the federal Centers for Disease Control and Prevention found 80 percent of adult Americans have at least one habit or condition that puts them at risk for heart disease. Check the statements that apply to you:

CATEGORY A: PRIMARY RISK FACTORS

1. My father (mother, brother or sister) has had heart disease. _____

2. My father (mother, brother or sister) had a heart attack before age fifty. _____

3. I'm a smoker. _____

4. I have high blood pressure (pressure over 140/90 mmHg). ____

5. My total blood cholesterol is above 240 mg/dl. _____

6. I am twenty lbs (or more) overweight. _____

7. I have diabetes. _____

CATEGORY B: SECONDARY RISK FACTORS

8. I seldom exercise. _____

9. I'm postmenopausal and I am not on hormone replacement therapy. _____

10. I smoke and take oral contraceptives. _____

11. I frequently eat red meat, full-fat dairy products, fast foods, snack foods, rich desserts. _____

12. I eat fewer than six daily servings of grains, five servings of vegetables and two servings of fruit a day. _____

13. I'm a heavy drinker (more than two to three drinks per day). _____

14. I use cocaine or other addictive drugs. _____

If you checked one or more primary risk factors in Category A, you could be at increased risk of cardiovascular disease and need to consult a physician. If you also checked one or more of the statements in Category B, factors in your lifestyle may be adding to your risk and may need to be changed.

WHAT WE KNOW ABOUT
WOMEN AND HEART DISEASE

The female hormone estrogen, which regulates ovulation and menstruation, seems to protect women against developing heart disease until after menopause. Women tend to get their first symptoms seven to ten years later than men, suffering heart attacks in their sixties, while men may start showing signs of cardiac disease in their forties and fifties.

When heart disease hits women, it hits hard and fast. Since women are much older, they get much sicker than men, and are more likely to die of heart disease. During the year after a heart attack, a woman's chances of a second attack are about 20 percent, compared with 16 percent for men. Women are also more prone to having strokes after a heart attack.

Much of this information about women and heart disease has come from the Framingham Heart Study, a prevention and treatment project that has followed the health of almost six thousand citizens of Framingham, Massachusetts, since 1948. It's the world's longest-running study of cardiovascular disease, and one of the few to include women in numbers equal to men; 1,930 daughters of the original participants are now being followed.

Vital new information has also come from the Nurses' Health Study, an ongoing research project at Harvard since 1976, which is examining a variety of risk factors among different groups (or "cohorts") among more than 121,000 registered nurses around the country. Among other things, this study showed the adverse effects of a high-fat diet and smoking on women's hearts.

In addition, the National Institutes of Health has been following the health of 5,115 men and women (half of whom are black) in Birmingham (Alabama), Chicago, Minneapolis and Oakland (California), to observe the evolution of risk factors and how they are affected by the lifestyles of young adults. The Coronary Artery Risk Development in Young Adults (CARDIA for short) is one of the largest such studies being conducted among African Americans. These are all important studies and we'll be referring to both of them a great deal throughout this book.

By far, the most significant lesson learned from all of these studies is that *heart disease can be prevented*. Over the past decade, prevention has helped reduce the death rate from coronary heart disease by 29 percent among women. But far too many women are still dying. Since 1984, female deaths from cardiovascular disease have continually surpassed male deaths.

THE HEART OF THE MATTER: HORMONES

A look at how men and women evolved since prehistoric times partly explains why women are less likely to get heart disease during their child-bearing years.

At puberty, a surge in the male hormone testosterone helps boys build muscle mass and carry more oxygen in the blood—traits that primitive man needed for survival in caveman days. While levels of blood cholesterol rise to help build muscles, levels of the "good" cholesterol, *high-density lipoprotein*, or *HDL*, which helps rid the body of excess blood fats, start to fall. The female hormone estrogen helps initiate biological changes to prepare girls for the future demands of pregnancy and nurturing a fetus. Estrogen boosts HDL in girls, while the "bad" cholesterol, *low-density lipoprotein*, or *LDL*, does not increase.

When men stop building muscle mass and become less active in middle age, theoretically, the unneeded LDL cholesterol ends up in their bloodstream. This speeds up *atherosclerosis*, the process in which fatty deposits narrow coronary arteries. Lacking a woman's "hormonal protection," to remove this excess blood fat, men become vulnerable to heart attacks in their forties.

In contrast, while estrogen is still being produced in her body, a woman is shielded from many of the factors that cause heart disease. Women accumulate fatty deposits in their arteries, but at a much slower rate. Take away estrogen, and the picture drastically changes. Women who undergo premature menopause or have their ovaries removed before age forty, for example, have a threefold increase in their risk of coronary disease.

For most women, estrogen production tapers off gradually until it ceases around the age of fifty, so heart disease tends to come on more gradually. Levels of HDL start to fall, allowing LDL cholesterol to increase, accelerating atherosclerosis. Total cholesterol levels rise and eventually surpass those of men.

In addition, the Framingham Offspring Study indicates that premenopausal women may have more of a natural clot buster circulating in their blood.

The cumulative result: Women start having heart attacks in the same numbers as men do—just a decade or so later.

But there's another "female advantage" in coronary disease that's often overlooked: Since women do get sick later than men, they also have *extra time to do something about risk factors that can be changed, and to prevent existing heart disease from getting worse.*

ADDING UP THE RISK EQUATION

While men and women share the same risk factors for heart disease, some factors pose a bigger threat for women:

Diabetes: This is a disease that impairs the body's ability to process blood sugar. It can damage blood vessels and lead to high blood pressure, kidney damage and kidney failure, as well as accelerate clogging of the arteries. Heart disease is the leading cause of death among people with diabetes, and women with diabetes are more than three times more likely to die of heart disease than diabetic men. As many as fourteen million Americans have some form of diabetes, and it is more common among women.

Smoking: New research indicates that the chemicals in cigarette smoke counteract the cardio-protective effects of estrogen. In addition, women who smoke experience menopause earlier than nonsmokers, and cigarette smoke also damages their arteries, making them more prone to blockages.

Smoking also increases a woman's risk of strokes, especially women taking birth control pills. About one quarter of American women smoke, and over the past thirty years, there's been a 45 percent increase in smoking in women over age sixty-five.

Race and Risk: Women of color, especially black women, are at increased risk of heart attacks. Data presented at a 1994 American Heart Association conference on heart disease in African-American women shows that death rates from cardiovascular disease among black women are 69 percent higher than for whites. Deaths from heart attacks among black women ages thirty-five to seventy-four are twice as high as those of white women, and three times greater than for women of other races; the rate among Native-American women is five times that of white women.

While about one fourth of women of all races have hypertension, the prevalence is 1.7 times higher in black women and rises to 73 percent between the ages of sixty-five and seventy-four. Over half of black women between ages twenty and seventy-four have borderline high or high cholesterol; blacks tend to have less of the "good" cholesterol than whites. The rate of diabetes among black women is twice as high as among white women; diabetes is also more common among Native-American women, and the numbers increase with age.

Almost 44 percent of black women in this country are overweight, compared with about one quarter of white women. All of these risk factors interact, with obesity leading to more diabetes and hypertension at an early age.

Poverty: Poverty and lack of access to medical care increase risk for women of all races. A 1993 review of forty years of research into heart disease found that better-educated and affluent Americans are less likely than poor people to die of heart disease and stroke.

Women ages forty-five to sixty-four, just at the age when they're entering the danger zone for heart attacks, are less likely to have health insurance than men. As many as 14 percent of American women have no health insurance and the rates are even higher among black and Latina women.* Latinos have the worst health coverage of any ethnic group in the United States, with 39 percent of those under age sixty-five having

_____
* Editor's Note: We have elected to use the term "Latina" to refer to women of Hispanic or Spanish-speaking background (including Puerto Rican Americans, Cuban Americans, Mexican Americans, and Latin Americans).

little or no health insurance. That's more than three times higher than whites and twice the rate of blacks. In addition, women of all races are more likely to be widowed and poorer by the time heart disease shows itself.

Experts hope that the adoption of universal health coverage in the future will improve this picture, especially since prevention (like cholesterol screening) will receive new emphasis.

The Effects of Gender: A flood of studies since 1987 have indicated that some women are not being adequately diagnosed and treated for coronary heart disease.

Studies indicate that many doctors have been too quick to dismiss women's symptoms as being psychological, and too slow to refer them for key diagnostic tests.

The problem is compounded even further because some of those tests can be less accurate in women. An exercise stress test, which measures heart activity during strenuous exercise, has a higher error rate in women. A woman's breast tissue may make it harder to get a clear picture of the heart during some radiological tests.

Women who are correctly diagnosed often receive less aggressive treatment than men. Fully 73 percent of bypass patients are men; a majority of angioplasty and heart transplants are also done in men.

Even when women *do* get the best care available, they often suffer more complications than men and die more often in the hospital after *angioplasty* (a procedure to open clogged coronary arteries) and coronary bypass surgery. One reason is that they are older and sicker when diagnosed.

Female Physiology: In addition to being older, most female heart patients have other health problems such as high blood pressure or diabetes. But even after allowing for those factors, statistics show that women *still* fare worse than men.

Since a woman's body mass is usually smaller than a man's, the coronary arteries supplying blood and oxygen to the heart are also smaller and narrower, which may mean they are more easily clogged by cholesterol deposits and may be more difficult to work with surgically.

Women may also have more clot-forming substances in their blood, leading to lessened reactions to clot-busting (or *thrombolytic*) medications. Reports in this country and in Europe found that when men and women were treated with the same thrombolytic drugs within four hours of a heart attack, women were twice as likely to die as men, and were more likely to suffer another heart attack within a year.

The reasons for this are unknown. Up until a few years ago, there were few (if any) clinical studies on why treatments affect men and women differently, what effect hormone therapy has on cardiovascular drugs, and how a woman's anatomy and body chemistry affect her chances of surviving a heart attack.

Add it all up and what you get is a clearly higher risk for women (especially women of color, poor women and older women), compounded by a lack of knowledge of just what to do about it.

WHERE WE STAND TODAY

Fortunately, the catch-up process has already begun.

The Women's Health Initiative (WHI), the largest study of women's health ever undertaken in the United States, is now under way. This landmark randomized clinical trial is aimed at reducing rates of heart disease, breast cancer, and osteoporosis. Some sixty thousand women ages fifty to seventy-nine are expected to take part in the trial, funded by the National Institutes of Health; one out of every five will be women of color.

Over the next fifteen years, the WHI hopes to find out whether estrogen replacement, estrogen and progesterone therapy, a low-fat diet and vitamin D and calcium supplements—singly or in combination—can reduce the incidence of heart disease.

NIH will also follow 100,000 women as they age in a long-range study aimed at improving risk prediction in heart disease, breast cancer and osteoporosis. The study will create a source of data that can be used to identify new risk factors and biomarkers for these diseases.

Researchers at Harvard Medical School and its teaching affiliate, Brigham and Women's Hospital in Boston, have begun a similar primary prevention trial, which will last at least five years. The randomized trial will involve forty thousand healthy, postmenopausal female health professionals to see if low-dose aspirin, beta carotene and vitamin E (singly or in combination with one another) can prevent heart disease (or cancer, or both).

Data from the first nationwide controlled clinical trial of hormone replacement, the Post-Menopausal Estrogen and Progestin Intervention

(PEPI) Trial are now being analyzed. The preliminary results, released late in 1994, appear in Chapter 10.

Another important step to improving women's overall medical care was taken in 1993. The U.S. Food and Drug Administration lifted its ban on women in drug safety tests; women had been excluded because of fears that drugs might affect an undiagnosed pregnancy. Drug studies must now include women and must find out if drugs affect women differently. In the past, as many as *half* of all cardiac drug studies did not include women or failed to look at gender differences. An office of women's health has also been set up at the FDA. The federal Centers for Disease Control and Prevention has established a similar office to coordinate its women's health programs.

The American Heart Association has also issued a new Scientific Statement on Women and Cardiovascular Disease, summarizing new information on risk factors and treatment. The statement puts forth new recommendations on oral contraceptives, hormone-replacement therapy and the use of aspirin after strokes, all of which are included in this book.

While more doctors *are* better informed these days about women and heart disease, it will take a decade or more to get results from new research that can be applied to treatment in women.

What can women do in the meantime?

We can start by taking control of our health, becoming as informed as possible about heart disease risk factors and prevention strategies. We need to know how symptoms may present themselves differently in women, what tests and treatments are available, as well as their risks and benefits, so that we can obtain the best medical care possible if there is a problem.

HOW YOUR CARDIOVASCULAR
SYSTEM WORKS

Your heart is an extraordinarily strong and sophisticated pump made of muscle, slightly bigger than your fist, with its own internal electrical system to keep it beating properly. A woman's heart is slightly smaller than a man's, but it pumps just as powerfully.

Each day, the heart beats (expands and contracts) an average of one hundred thousand times and pumps almost two thousand gallons of blood rich in oxygen and nutrients through a vast network of blood vessels to all the organs and tissues of the body. These blood vessels include arteries, smaller arteries called arterioles, and capillaries.

Parts of the Heart

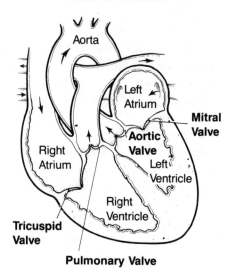

"Heart Valve Surgery," 1991,
copyright © American Heart
Association. Reprinted by
permission.

In the capillaries, carbon dioxide and waste materials are collected in the blood from organs and tissues, then circulated back to the heart through another network of blood vessels (including veins and *venules*, or small veins). These waste products are filtered out as blood passes through the lungs, kidneys and liver.

The heart has four chambers. The two upper chambers of the heart are called *atria*, the two lower chambers are called *ventricles*. There are valves between each chamber with flaps (also called *cuspids* or *leaflets*) that open and close to make sure blood flows in the right direction and doesn't back up into the chamber which it's just exited.

The sequence goes like this:

• The right atrium admits blood from two large veins, the superior vena cava and the inferior vena cava.

• While the heart is relaxed, venous blood flows through the open tricuspid valve to fill the right ventricle.

• An electrical impulse is sent to the right atrium to contract. This "tops off" the filling of the right ventricle.

• The right ventricle contracts, shutting the tricuspid valve and opening the pulmonary valve, shooting blood through the pulmonary artery into the lungs.

• In the lungs, waste products are removed and fresh oxygen is put into blood, giving it the familiar bright red color.

• Oxygenated blood leaves the lungs, passing through the pulmonary vein into the left atrium, where it's sent through the mitral valve into the left ventricle.

• The left ventricle contracts, closing the mitral valve and pumping the blood into the aorta, out to the organs and tissues.

What Makes a Heart Beat

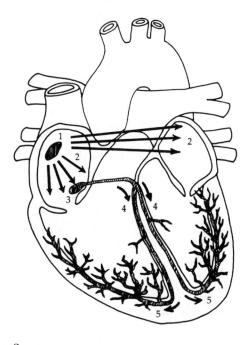

Source:
National Heart,
Lung and Blood
Institute.

The trigger for this sequence of events is an electrical impulse originating in a small group of highly specialized cells in the right atrium, the *sinoatrial node* (or SA) (1).

The impulse moves through the right and left atria (2), is transmitted to the *atrioventricular node* (3) and then down specialized nerve fibers in the ventricles (4, 5), causing them to contract in almost a wringing motion, squeezing out blood.

The first organ that gets fed in this circulatory process is actually the heart itself, when oxygen-rich blood flows through the coronary arteries.

THINGS THAT CAN GO WRONG

Atherosclerosis: In atherosclerosis, excess cholesterol in the blood accumulates in fatty *plaques* inside the coronary arteries, making the inner wall of the vessel, or *lumen*, progressively smaller so less blood flows through. Atherosclerosis can also occur in blood vessels in the kidneys, legs, or neck.

An estimated fifty-five million adult women in this country have blood cholesterol above the 200 milligrams per deciliter of blood that's considered healthy. More than 60 percent of white women and 54 percent of African-American women fall into this group.

Ischemia/Angina: When blood flow to the heart is severely restricted, it causes a condition called *ischemia*. Ischemia may trigger pain in heart muscle cells because they are not getting enough blood to meet their needs. This chest pressure or pain is called *angina pectoris*, and it is usually the *first* symptom of coronary artery disease.

More than three million people in America suffer from angina, with three hundred fifty thousand new cases a year, many of them women. In general, women are almost twice as likely as men to suffer angina (but the prevalence is almost the same for black men and women). *Unstable angina*, in which symptoms occur without exertion or follow a predictable pattern, is much more common among women.

Some women have ischemia without any chest pain at all, a condition aptly called *silent ischemia*. Some of these women may suffer a heart attack with no warning. Diabetics may be especially prone to silent ischemia.

Heart Attacks: If blood flow to part of the heart is restricted for more than thirty minutes or is blocked completely, that part of the heart muscle will begin to die. That's what happens in a heart attack, or a *myocardial infarction*.

Almost half of the 500,000 heart attack deaths in this country every year are women. While 5 percent of heart attacks occur in people under age forty, the number rises to 45 percent before age sixty-five. At older ages, women are twice as likely as men to die within a few weeks of suffering a heart attack. By age sixty-five and over, deaths from ischemic heart disease are 11 percent higher for women than for men.

High Blood Pressure: Life-threatening problems can also occur when the heart must work harder than normal to pump blood through the body's network of blood vessels.

Healthy blood vessels stretch with each spurt of blood that occurs when the heart beats. Damaged blood vessels lose this flexibility or, for a variety of reasons, they constrict instead of expanding. This causes resistance to blood flow, which then forces a rise in blood pressure.

When blood pressure is constantly elevated over a normal level it is known as *hypertension.* Untreated hypertension strains the heart and blood vessels and can contribute to heart attacks, strokes, kidney failure and atherosclerosis. The heart may also enlarge and the blood vessels become scarred.

After age forty-five, 60 percent of white women and 79 percent of black women have hypertension. African-American, Latina and Native-American women are most at risk for high blood pressure. Some 35 percent of people with hypertension don't even know they have it; only about 21 percent are adequately controlling it.

Strokes: Most commonly, an artery supplying blood to the brain, narrowed by atherosclerotic plaques, becomes blocked by a blood clot, causing an *ischemic stroke.*

Heart-rhythm abnormalities can also lead to formation of blood clots in the heart, which can travel to the brain, causing an *embolic stroke.* Chronic high blood pressure may weaken blood vessels in the brain, causing them to burst, resulting in a *hemorrhagic stroke.*

Ischemic strokes are often preceded by a "ministroke" or *transient ischemic attack* (TIA), which causes faintness, temporary loss of speech or sight in one eye and temporary weakness in one side of the body. A recent study indicates that these ministrokes may be responsible for many preventable and treatable cases of *senile dementia* among older women, which may otherwise be diagnosed as Alzheimer's disease.

The American Heart Association says strokes claim more than eighty-seven thousand lives among women each year, more than 60 percent of all stroke fatalities. Of women who survive a stroke, 61 percent suffer some sort of permanent disability.

Because of the high rates of hypertension in the African-American community, blacks are twice as likely as whites to suffer a stroke, often with more severity and at a much younger age. The death rate for stroke among black women is almost 80 percent higher than among white women.

Congestive Heart Failure: Congestive heart failure is different from a heart attack in that the heart muscle is not acutely damaged; it just has trouble keeping up with the demands of the body. The heart pumps so weakly that it fails to pump enough blood to the kidneys, causing a buildup of fluids in the tissues, which leads to extreme fatigue and shortness of breath.

Heart failure may result from a number of things, including damage from a heart attack or heart enlargement due to chronic high blood pressure, heart valve disease, or alcohol and drug abuse.

It's estimated that 2.3 to 3 million Americans, most of them older adults, are living with congestive heart failure, with 400,000 new cases diagnosed every year. Approximately half of people who suffer congestive heart failure are women. It is the leading cause of death and hospitalization after age sixty-five.

Cardiac Arrhythmias: When the heart is severely diseased, or when one of its electrical pathways is blocked by scar tissue from a heart attack, other parts of the heart rather than the sinoatrial node may be forced to generate a heartbeat. The result is a potentially dangerous slowed or irregular heartbeat, called a *cardiac arrhythmia* (or *dysrhythmia*). In some cases, cardiac arrhythmia can cause sudden death.

Almost four million Americans have some form of cardiac arrhythmia. Drug abuse, especially cocaine, has become an increasing cause of arrhythmias in young people in recent years.

All told, more than half the deaths each year among white women occur as a result of heart and blood vessel diseases, and the percentage is even higher among African-American women. The death rate is about 40 percent among Asian-Pacific Islander women, about 37 percent for Latina women and 32 percent for Native-American women.

HOW YOU CAN
CHANGE YOUR RISK

Some risk factors for heart disease can't be changed, of course. We can't stop the aging process or change the families or racial groups we were born into. Simply having a mother, father or sibling who suffered a heart attack before age fifty increases your risk of heart disease five to ten times.

But women *can* and should do something about those risk factors that are changeable.

According to the American Heart Association Scientific Statement on Women and Cardiovascular Disease, the three most important behaviors that can prevent heart disease among women are: avoid smoking; eat a balanced, low-saturated-fat diet to control blood fats and maintain a moderate level of physical activity to help control weight. These three steps will also keep blood pressure in check and control or prevent diabetes.

If you act *now*, you'll make some big gains:

• Quitting smoking reduces a woman's coronary risk by 50 to 70 percent.

• Reducing high blood pressure can cut the risk of heart disease by 15 to 20 percent.

• Lowering cholesterol can mean a 20 to 30 percent drop in heart attack rates.

• Avoiding obesity by losing weight could cut your risk of heart disease by 35 to 50 percent.

• Exercising regularly will reduce your risk by 45 percent.

None of us is perfect. We may be aware of what's healthful and what isn't, but we encounter hurdles that prevent us from taking action. Some have to do with the way we were raised; some have to do with the kind of life we lead. Other hurdles are just piles of excuses that get too high to climb over.

We hope that the recommendations in this book will help you get over the hurdles that stand between awareness and action.

Each chapter has been prepared under the careful technical guidance of physicians and other health professionals at New York University Medical Center, NYU's Women's Health Service and the Division of Cardiology. We've also talked with leading experts to gather the very latest information on women and heart disease; some of this material is very new and still under study, but has been carefully reviewed by the researchers involved.

This book contains the updated federal guidelines for the prevention and treatment of high blood pressure and high cholesterol. In addition, you'll get the benefit of NYU's Weight Management Program for Women to help you acquire better eating habits or lose those extra pounds, and the Smokeless self-help program to help you kick the habit if you're a smoker.

This book will explain what symptoms of cardiovascular disease typically feel like in women, so you'll be more likely to recognize them if they do occur.

Also provided is information on diagnostic tests (and when they may be indicated); treatments for heart problems; and special issues of concern to women in the recovery process.

We'll provide an understanding of the latest thinking on gender bias in the treatment of heart disease, as well as advice on choosing and communicating effectively with physicians.

Every effort also has been made to make this book multicultural, addressing the questions, needs and problems facing women of different backgrounds. Throughout this book you'll hear the voices of different women, sharing their experiences about everything from quitting smoking to recovering from heart surgery (names and identifying factors have been changed to protect their privacy).

Appendix III provides a list of organizations that can provide more information and direct you to top cardiology facilities and support groups in your area. Appendix IV offers a selected listing of recent books on heart disease and related health issues, and low-fat cookbooks.

Avoiding heart disease means taking steps to safeguard your health *now*. We hope that this book will help you to do just that.

2

Clearing the Smoke Screen

OF ALL THE preventable risk factors for heart disease, smoking tops the list. Nearly one fifth of deaths from cardiovascular disease can be attributed to smoking. A woman who smokes has a two to six times greater risk of a heart attack than a nonsmoker, and smoking is *far worse* for women than for men.

According to the Framingham Heart Study, a woman smoker has a 15 percent higher risk of heart attacks than a male smoker. If she has other risk factors, such as high blood pressure or high cholesterol, her risk is 20 to 30 percent higher than that of a man who smokes.

The latest research says that *smoking actually robs a woman of her hormonal protection against heart disease by contributing to an earlier menopause* and causing heart disease among women as young as in their twenties or thirties.

The *good* news is that when you quit, you start to cancel out tobacco's negative cardiac effects. Within a few years, your risk of a heart attack will be the same as a woman who's never smoked! You can actually *add* several years to your life by quitting.

You may have tried to kick the habit several times before and couldn't do it. Perhaps you found the pleasure of smoking outweighed warnings about its perils, or maybe you were afraid you'd gain weight.

To get over these hurdles, you need to understand the real reasons why you smoke, and find realistic and effective ways to help yourself stay off cigarettes. You also need to comprehend fully what each one of those cigarettes is really doing to your body.

WHAT SMOKING DOES
TO YOUR BODY

After a slight decline in recent years, more women are now smoking. The most recent figures from the Centers for Disease Control and Prevention show that some 23 million American women smoke, an increase of almost 1 percent.

Smoking even just a few cigarettes a day can put your risk of dying from coronary disease up to 67 percent higher than a nonsmoker's. A woman who smokes two packs of cigarettes a day is likely to have a heart attack eleven years earlier than a nonsmoker. For African-American women, smoking-related disorders such as high blood pressure and stroke are more severe than in white women.

The chemicals in cigarette smoke progressively poison the entire cardiovascular system in the following ways:

• Scientists in the United States, Italy and Sweden found that smoking decreases normal estrogen production. Since estrogen helps keep cholesterol levels lower, this may be why female smokers tend to have higher cholesterol. Smoking also increases the amount of male hormones in women (normally present in very small amounts), which also tends to lower levels of "good" HDL cholesterol. And smoking raises levels of a blood fat called *triglycerides* that depletes levels of HDL.

• Women who smoke undergo menopause as much as five years earlier (at about age forty-seven) than nonsmoking women, and this places them at risk for heart disease earlier in life. In addition, menopausal symptoms such as hot flashes are aggravated in smokers. (Chemicals in cigarette smoke also appear to speed the bone-wasting disease osteoporosis as well as slow healing of fractures caused by brittle bones.)

• Carbon monoxide in cigarette smoke immediately endangers the heart. According to Stanton Glantz, Ph.D., a smoking researcher at the University of California at San Francisco (UCSF), carbon monoxide competes with oxygen for space in red blood cells, reducing the blood's ability to carry oxygen. In addition, animal tests show that the oxygen that gets transported to the heart isn't converted to energy as efficiently.

• Carbon monoxide and other chemicals in smoke damage or irritate the inner walls of coronary arteries, causing tiny cracks where excess fats in the blood can accumulate. Smokers have a distinctive kind of atherosclerotic lesion not found in nonsmokers.

• A 1993 update from the Nurses' Health Study found that women who smoked forty-five or more cigarettes a day were five times more at risk for stroke than nonsmokers.

• Tobacco smoke contains chemicals that make blood platelets get stickier, so stroke and heart-attack-causing blood clots may occur. Women smokers also have been found to have higher levels of *fibrinogen*, needed for blood clotting after an injury. Increased levels of fibrinogen are associated with higher than normal rates of coronary artery disease.

• The clotting risk is even worse for women who smoke and take oral contraceptives. Women on the pill who smoke are up to thirty-nine times more likely to have a heart attack and twenty-two times more likely to suffer a stroke than women who neither smoked nor took the pill.

• Smoking leads to high blood pressure. Nicotine signals the brain to produce the stress hormone adrenaline. Adrenaline makes the heart beat faster, which may cause irregular heart rhythms and constrict blood vessels, leading to hypertension. Scientists at the University of Iowa say coronary arteries contract by up to 38 percent for a half hour after each cigarette.

• Women smokers are more likely to use cigarettes to relieve stress or depression, yet a 1992 report from the Iowa Heart Institute in Des Moines found that smoking only makes these things *worse*! During times of physical and emotional stress, blood flow through tiny blood vessels called arterioles that feed the heart was found to be 30 percent less in smokers, due to previously unsuspected damage from smoking. Blood flow was decreased even when the person was not smoking and went down by another 20 percent once they lit up. Even scarier, this damage does *not* show up on conventional heart tests.

• Passive smoking hurts your heart, too. Dr. Glantz and his research team report that nonsmokers who live or work with smokers are 30 percent more likely to die of heart disease. Secondhand smoke causes between thirty-seven thousand and forty thousand deaths from heart disease among *nonsmokers* every year. In fact, according to UCSF's research, non-smokers seem to be more sensitive to the effects of cigarette smoke on their heart and blood vessels than smokers. Secondhand smoke makes women who already have heart problems more prone to angina and heart rhythm disturbances during physical exertion.

All of this does not even take into account smoking-related respiratory diseases like emphysema or asthma, which also have dangerous effects on the cardiovascular systems. Lung cancer kills more women every year than breast cancer, and smoking has also recently been linked to cervical cancer, which primarily kills poor women in America.

WHAT QUITTING DOES
FOR YOUR HEART

If you ditch those cigarettes right now, your health will improve almost immediately.

Within twenty minutes, your blood pressure and pulse rate will drop to the levels they were before you lit up. Within eight hours, your blood levels of carbon monoxide and oxygen will return to normal. Other toxic chemicals will clear from your lungs and bloodstream. Within seventy-two hours, you'll be breathing easier because your lung capacity will have increased.

If you stay off cigarettes indefinitely, you'll also cancel out most of the long-term health risks of smoking. A 1994 update from the Nurses' Health Study found that quitting smoking resulted in a one-third reduction in the risk of heart disease within two years, and smoking-related excess heart risk disappeared entirely within ten to fourteen years. Data from the Nurses' Health Study also found that quitting decreases a woman's risk of stroke *almost completely* within two to four years.

But don't think that switching to so-called "lite" or low-tar filtered cigarettes is a substitute for quitting. The Boston University scientists say smoking low-tar brands carries the *same* risk of heart attack as smoking regular cigarettes. There's also evidence that the paper on filtered cigarettes is not as porous as paper used on regular brands, so you end up inhaling more smoke. People who switch to low-tar cigarettes may also inhale more deeply (and thus actually smoke more).

The *only* way to reduce your risk is to quit completely—and quit for good.

WHY DO WOMEN SMOKE?

The decline in smoking during the past twenty-five years seems to have come to a halt, despite the much-publicized health risks and ever-widening public smoking restrictions. About one fourth of women over age eighteen now smoke.

According to the federal Centers for Disease Control and Prevention, Native-American/Native-Alaskan women smoke more than any other group (more than 35 percent), compared with 24.4 percent of black women and 23.8 percent of white women. Among Asian/Pacific Islander women, 7.5 percent smoke, compared with 15.5 percent of Latina women.

The tendency to smoke varies among Latino groups; 10 percent more Puerto Rican–American women smoke than women of Mexican or Cuban origin. In traditional Latino families, smoking is seen as something only men should do; women aren't supposed to drink or smoke, especially in public. So for some Latina women, smoking is a sign of "liberation."

Among African-American women, there was an overall increase of about 3 percent in the number of smokers. Interestingly, however, the rates of smoking among black women aged eighteen to twenty-four showed a sharp decline between 1991 and 1992, while smoking increased among white women in that age group. Cigarettes are being aggressively marketed in minority communities, with sponsorship of concerts or sports, huge billboards and clothing premiums.

While two million women quit smoking in 1993, teenage smoking increased. Cigarette advertising apparently has an enormous influence on impressionable young girls. A 1994 study in the *Journal of the American Medical Association* found a sharp increase in the number of girls ages ten to seventeen who began smoking in the late 1960s and early 1970s, when so-called "women's cigarettes" like Virginia Slims and Eve were introduced. Between 1967 and 1973, when sales of such brands hit $16 billion, there was a 110 percent increase in the number of twelve-year-old girls who started smoking! Those teenage girls who started smoking in the 1960s are now approaching their menopausal years, the danger zone for heart disease.

The latest figures show that three thousand young people start smoking every day (even though sales of cigarettes to minors are illegal). The National Institute of Education says teenage girls are five times more likely to smoke if one or both of their parents or an older sibling smokes. Teenage girls are more likely than boys to start smoking as a way to gain peer approval. People who have only a high-school education or who dropped out of high school are five times more likely to smoke than those with more education.

ALLYCE'S STORY

"I've smoked since I was thirteen; I'm twenty-six now. My mother is a smoker and she did try to discourage me. She said she didn't know it was so dangerous when she was young. I guess I started out smoking because I thought it was cool and made me look older. It was definitely peer pressure. I don't think I'm addicted to nicotine, but I'm psychologically hooked. My husband smokes, too.

"When I found out I was pregnant, I gave up smoking immediately because I heard it was bad for the baby. I was really good, too, until Sarah was about three months old. I had left my job, I was alone at home, we were having money problems, the baby was fussy, my husband was working nights, and I was just so up-tight. I'd go out on the back steps to take a few puffs just to relax. Before I knew it, I was back to a pack a day. We both know it's a bad habit and we try not to smoke around the baby.

"My mom just had a heart attack, and she's only fifty-five; that scares me. She's never been sick a day in her life, and suddenly, she's in Intensive Care. . . . Her doctor says she has to quit smoking or it will happen again. I guess we all have to quit. I mean, what if it happened to me? Or my husband? What if we made Sarah sick? But it's going to be hard, really hard."

Studies show that one of the most common reasons why young women start smoking is weight control. Cigarettes do depress appetite, may help the body burn more calories and are an oral substitute for food. In fact, way back in 1928, a cigarette ad advised women: "Reach for a Lucky Instead of a Sweet." Many "women's" cigarettes use the words *thin* or *slim* as part of the brand name.

Unrealistic standards of female slenderness contribute to yo-yo dieting, excessive use of diet pills and eating disorders, as well as to women smoking as a means of losing weight.

"Once smoking becomes a way of keeping weight down, many women become afraid they won't be able to control their food intake and fear they'll gain huge amounts of weight if they quit smoking," notes Nanette K. Wenger, M.D., a professor of medicine in cardiology and expert on women's health issues at Emory University in Atlanta.

Actually, only a third of people who quit smoking gain weight, and most women on average gain only five pounds or less after quitting smoking. Some women experience temporary weight gain because their metabolisms may have been abnormally elevated by cigarettes (especially if they were heavy smokers).

"For many women, even five extra pounds around the hips is perceived as an enormous weight gain. So women have to be extra careful about eating habits when they quit smoking," Dr. Wenger advises. If they seek out an organized smoking cessation program, it should offer help in eating behaviors, adoption of exercise, lifestyle modifications, and developing a positive body image.

But there's good news. One recent study from Canada found that although women do gain weight in the first year or so after quitting, afterward, most female smokers lose those extra pounds. The study also found that two years after kicking the habit, the ex-smokers were *less* likely to be obese than smokers!

If you do gain a pound or two, remember: According to the American Lung Association, you'd have to gain *fifty pounds* to put the equivalent strain on your heart that smoking does!

The worst thing to do is attempt a weight-loss diet while trying to quit smoking. Instead, Dr. Wenger advises women to be more aware of when they are eating to cope with nicotine withdrawal or stress, and to make sure they have plenty of low-calorie snacks on hand. Exercise can boost metabolism, is a substantial help in preventing weight gain and can aid in reducing stress at the same time.

A small preliminary study by the Center for Pulmonary Disease Prevention in Palo Alto, California, found that chewing two- or four-milligram doses of nicotine gum every hour during the day for a month helped a group of women who quit smoking keep weight gain to less than a pound. Curiously, the men didn't get the same benefit. However, experts caution, it could have been the act of chewing the gum, not the gum itself, that prevented weight gain.

UNDERSTANDING NICOTINE ADDICTION

According to the National Institute on Drug Abuse, nicotine is as addictive as heroin and five to ten times more potent than cocaine in its effects on mood and behavior!

Inhale on a cigarette and in about ten seconds, the nicotine goes from the lungs to the brain. There it hits the cerebral cortex, our center of reasoning, where it improves cognitive performance, stimulates alertness and triggers feelings of pleasure and satisfaction.

Researchers at the University of South Florida at Tampa say nicotine and other cigarette chemicals may react more strongly in women, increasing their craving and making it harder for them to quit smoking. In fact, some 77 percent of smokers want to quit but find it hard, mostly because of nicotine addiction!

During congressional hearings in 1994, the U.S. Food and Drug Administration charged that tobacco companies had increased the amount of nicotine in cigarettes to keep smokers addicted and added other compounds to increase the delivery of nicotine, charges the tobacco industry denied. However, the FDA is considering having cigarettes classified and regulated as addictive drugs.

The U.S. Department of Health says that women are more likely than men to turn to nicotine when under stress or in situations characterized by negative or unpleasant emotions like anger (which women are socially conditioned to suppress). Suppressing anger may be a behavioral risk factor for heart disease (see page 146), and smoking only adds to the damage.

People prone to depression may also have a hard time staying off cigarettes. Since nicotine boosts their mood, they are 25 percent more likely to become seriously depressed when they quit smoking; their success rate in smoking cessation programs is only about 6 percent. For such people, psychotherapy and antidepressants may hold the key to breaking their nicotine addiction.

Studies suggest that smokers who light up right after awakening may be among the most addicted to nicotine and may be good candidates for nicotine replacement. According to 1994 American Medical Association guidelines for treating nicotine dependence, other good candidates are people who smoke more than twenty cigarettes a day; those who smoke when ill or who find it hard not to smoke where it is forbidden; and those who had withdrawal symptoms during earlier attempts to quit.

MARGERY'S STORY

"I'm forty-eight and I just had a double bypass. I was never over-weight, I always ate healthy and I was pretty active. But I was a smoker for thirty years. I smoked a pack of cigarettes a day.

"I started when I was seventeen or eighteen. When I started smok-ing, no one ever said it was bad for your health. Everyone I knew smoked. I got addicted to the nicotine.

"I remember a few years ago, when other people I knew were quitting because it was the healthy thing to do, I'd say, 'I'm going to stop, too.' But I never did. Until I wound up in the hospital with two coronary-artery blockages. Then I had no choice. I had to quit.

"I didn't believe how strong the drug addiction was until I stopped. I was amazed at the cravings I had. And the more I got back into my normal routine, months after my bypass, the worse the cravings were. After dinner, I would automatically reach for a pack of cigarettes that wasn't there. It used to drive me crazy.

"I would say to myself, 'Just one, I'll just have one.' And here I was just having gone through open-heart surgery! I knew it was a drug addiction and I'd have to fight it. So I'd say to myself: 'Not even one. Not any. Do you want to commit suicide?'

"I can't tell a smoker to give up smoking because I was a smoker and I know they're not going to give it up until they're ready. And that's it. I often feel angry that I can't smoke anymore. Doesn't that sound dumb? I guess I will always have a craving for cigarettes, like an alcoholic with liquor."

YES, YOU CAN
KICK THE HABIT

Stopping your intake of nicotine will have physical and psychological withdrawal symptoms. *Rest assured, the symptoms do go away.*

Physical symptoms can include intense cravings for a cigarette, irri-tability, restlessness, trouble concentrating or sleeping, headaches, fatigue, dizziness and even rapid heartbeat, says Eileen DiFrisco, R.N., senior nurse-educator at NYU Medical Center. These symptoms are generally worse within two to three days after you quit. For some people, the symp-toms may dissipate within a month; for others, it may take longer.

During the initial withdrawal period, it is very important to stay away from other smokers as much as possible, DiFrisco advises. Being around smokers may weaken your resolve. For many people, she notes, psychological withdrawal is the hardest.

Within forty-eight to seventy-two hours, the nicotine may be out of your system, but the urge to smoke may not. For those who are nicotine-dependent, there are a number of products that can ease withdrawal:

Nicotine Patches: Available by prescription only, transdermal nicotine patches are worn on the upper arm and gradually deliver a small dose of nicotine through the skin into the bloodstream over a twenty-four-hour period. Once you put a patch on, it takes about twenty minutes to half an hour to start working on nicotine receptors in the brain, satisfying the craving for cigarettes. A twenty-one-milligram nicotine patch delivers the equivalent amount of nicotine over a day contained in approximately one pack of cigarettes. Some adhesive cloth patches are designed to be worn only during waking hours.

The 1994 AMA guidelines suggest that patch use begin on the quit date and continue for six to ten weeks. Nicotine patches work best as part of smoking cessation programs, using diminishing doses combined with behavior therapy. Patches must be changed every day and cost about one hundred twenty dollars per month for the three or four months it generally takes to wean a smoker off nicotine. Side effects can include insomnia and skin irritation, so the site is usually rotated.

A recent analysis of seventeen studies involving five thousand men and women smokers found that patch users were twice as likely to stay off cigarettes for six months, compared to those on placebo.

A warning for patch wearers: Don't smoke! There have been reports of heart attacks among some people who smoked while using nicotine patches. The U.S. Food and Drug Administration is investigating these cases.

Nicotine Gum: Prescription nicotine-replacement gum works on the same principle as the patch. Gum chewers must periodically park their wad of nicotine gum between the jaw and the cheek for a proper dose to be absorbed. Side effects include jaw aches as well as sore throats and hiccups. The gum costs about twenty-five dollars a week and may be used for as long as six months.

New reports suggest that coffee, cola and acidic foods like citrus fruit and fruit juice can interfere with absorption of nicotine in the gum. Experts advise avoiding drinking or eating anything but water for fifteen minutes before using nicotine gum.

Nicotine gum may soon be sold without prescription. The gum appears to be slightly less successful than the patch but, again, *neither keeps people off cigarettes indefinitely without some sort of support program.*

Hypnosis: Hypnosis can be done both in individual or group sessions. Treatment is usually one session of one to two hours, with special audiocassettes to reinforce the technique at home. The cost can range from $150 to $350 per session.

Studies have found that hypnosis helps 90 percent of participants quit, but only 10 to 15 percent stay off cigarettes longer than one year.

Acupuncture: Acupuncture for smoking cessation involves the placement of special needles in specific points of a person's earlobe. The process supposedly sends chemical messages through nerve endings to the brain to block nicotine cravings. It usually costs about fifty dollars per session; treatment usually involves four to six sessions lasting about half an hour. Unfortunately, acupuncture for smoking cessation has not yet been clinically tested for its long-term effectiveness.

Over-the-Counter Aids: Nonprescription stop-smoking aids include special filters and stop-smoking kits. Some of these filters gradually reduce the amount of tar and nicotine a person inhales. The problem is, the person is still smoking cigarettes while they're using the filters and they may end up smoking more in order to make up for the reduced nicotine effect.

Antidepressants: The antidepressant sertraline (Zoloft) is being tested in clinical trials to see if it helps depression-prone smokers kick the habit. Preliminary evidence shows the drug may have doubled the quit rate. Studies of the drug buproprion (Welbutrin), which appears to affect brain chemicals in ways similar to nicotine, are also being conducted.

As of December 1, 1993, the U.S. Food and Drug Administration banned the sale of other over-the-counter smoking deterrent products such as pills, tablets, lozenges and chewing gums, saying there's no proof that they work.

GROUP SUPPORT PROGRAMS

There are at least a dozen group support programs offered around the country to help you quit smoking.

Programs range from courses like SmokeEnders (often sponsored by corporations for their employees) to free, nonprofit programs such as Fresh Start, run by local chapters of the American Cancer Society. Most last one to two weeks, with additional support sessions available.

The federal Centers for Disease Control and Prevention in Atlanta (CDC) says that the *most* effective programs provide support groups, set a firm deadline for quitting, and offer nicotine gum or patches. Costs can range from twenty dollars for a nonprofit smoking cessation course to several hundred dollars for a clinical program, often with extra charges for nicotine patches, gum, stress-reduction exercise tapes, and other supplies.

Women should consider a smoking cessation program that has a strong dietary component, since weight control is a major issue in smoking. Look for a program at your local church, synagogue, or civic group. These programs are likely to be less expensive and you'll be closer to home. Babysitting may even be available.

You'll find just about every kind of quitting technique in use. Some programs use "aversion therapy," which can range from marathon puffing to mild electric shocks.

The Smokeless program offered at NYU Medical Center makes use of a technique called "negative smoking."

The Smokeless program was developed by the American Institute for Preventive Medicine and is run by specially trained professionals in corporate and hospital settings. It involves four consecutive group sessions of one and a half hours each over a week (or five hour-long sessions), plus three follow-up maintenance meetings. Its success rate is somewhat higher than other smoking cessation programs, with 65 percent of participants staying off cigarettes after a year. The program is also available as a self-help kit.

The idea behind "negative smoking" is to replace the chain of pleasant associations with smoking with unpleasant associations, especially the taste and smell of cigarettes. These unpleasant sensations can be recalled later on and used to help tame the urge to smoke.

In "negative smoking," participants are told to *puff* on cigarettes, rather than inhale them, causing a buildup of bitter-tasting nicotine on the tongue.

In one exercise, called digit dragging, participants are told to hold a cigarette in the opposite smoking hand, between their pinky and ring fingers, and puff on the cigarette from the opposite side of the mouth where they usually inhale. This results in accumulating too much smoke around the face and makes the lips feel hot. It also makes the participant feel awkward, as opposed to the smoothness of their accustomed smoking gestures.

While these puffing exercises are going on, the instructor rapidly flashes a sequence of slides showing the dire consequences of smoking, further reinforcing the negative associations, all the while stressing to the participants that they are in control and they can choose *not* to smoke.

For those quitters who don't even want to be around cigarette smoke, there are smoke-free negative smoking exercises. One makes use of a "butt bottle," where participants are asked to sniff a bottle filled with old ashes and cigarette butts while visualizing the unpleasant aspects of smoking.

"Negative smoking" is used for three days, while participants are also taught behavior and diet modification and various ways of handling stress, including positive thinking and mental imagery.

While programs like these are effective, the CDC says that about 90 percent of former smokers kicked the habit on their own, using self-help methods and free or low-cost pamphlets and kits available through organizations like the American Lung Association or the American Cancer Society. For *heavy* smokers, however, smoking cessation programs along with nicotine gum, patches or hypnosis were more effective, keeping 20 to 40 percent away from cigarettes for at least a year.

CAROL'S STORY

"I had tried quitting smoking I don't know how many times. What tripped me up each and every time was that I'd be ravenously hungry all day. I was always stuffing my face, so I'd gain a lot of weight. And I literally would panic when I looked at the scale and saw how fat I was getting.

"Until I joined 'Smokeless,' I never thought about why I was smoking. I thought it was just the weight thing. But I realized that I was like a baby with a security blanket. When I'd feel tense, I reached for a cigarette. When I was hungry, I'd reach for a cigarette. When I was out in a crowd, I'd light up and feel more relaxed. Even after our office went smoke-free, in the coldest weather there would be this bunch of us outside shivering taking a cigarette break. It was like a club, us against the world. Funny, how cigarettes became part of so many things in my life. The Smokeless program taught me to think about this kind of stuff each time I craved a smoke. Some of it seemed so stupid, looking back now.

"Quitting wasn't easy. But this time I just gained two pounds because they warned us to keep low-calorie foods around. You wouldn't believe how hard I chewed to fight the urge.

"I admit I was really motivated to quit for good this time because my fiancé doesn't smoke. He really hates it. That was a big part of it. But you know what really did the trick? Smelling that 'butt bottle' with the old cigarettes in it. It was so disgusting. My fiancé told me that's what my hair smelled like when I smoked."

GOING "SMOKELESS"

If you're going to try to quit on your own, here are six basic rules that have proven successful in the Smokeless program:

One: Set a target date for quitting and stick to it. Nurse-educator Eileen DiFrisco, who runs the Smokeless program at NYU Medical Center, says that for most people, quitting cold turkey is the best way to go. The longer you stay off cigarettes, the less you're likely to relapse. In fact, a 1994 study found that *total abstinence* during the first fourteen days of quitting was a strong predictor of success among people using nicotine patch therapy.

DiFrisco believes that gradually reducing the amount you smoke doesn't work, because the cigarettes you *do* smoke become more and more important as there are fewer and fewer of them, so it's harder to give up those precious last few smokes.

Two: Get rid of cigarettes you may have stashed away. If you have a secret supply in your car's glove compartment or in a desk drawer, dump it. Also get rid of ashtrays and smoking paraphernalia, including that fancy cigarette lighter you loved to flash. Don't just put them away, throw them away!

Three: Teach yourself to associate smoking with negative sensations and thoughts. DiFrisco recommends the "butt bottle" technique. When you're getting rid of your ashtrays, save the contents in a small bottle. Whenever you get the urge to smoke, take a whiff of this mess. Then picture dirty gray cigarette smoke going into your lungs, depositing a residue of cancer-causing chemicals and leaving a foul odor on your clothing, skin and furnishings. Sound yucky? It is.

Four: Consciously change smoking-related behavior. You probably have linked cigarettes with certain behaviors, such as smoking with a cup of coffee first thing in the morning or lighting up while you make a phone call. DiFrisco suggests "scrambling" those behaviors; instead of coffee, have orange juice; doodle while you're on the phone instead of smoking.

Consider keeping a smoking diary. When you get the urge to smoke, write down the circumstances and what you're feeling. Once you understand the behaviors and emotions involved with smoking, you can consciously work on changing them.

Five: Keep lots of low-calorie munchies on hand. Unbuttered popcorn, raw vegetables or sugarless mints can keep your mouth busy when the urge to light up strikes. It's important to remember that you won't turn into a blimp overnight unless you *overeat*. Turn that 1920s cigarette ad upside down: Reach for a carrot stick instead of a smoke.

Six: Learn some stress-management techniques. See Chapter 8 for helpful techniques. If you learn other ways of handling stress, you won't need the calming effects of nicotine.

Exercise is a perfect stress-buster *and* waistline tamer. Exercise also has antidepressant effects; you may find you'll get the same emotional lift from a brisk walk that you used to get from a cigarette!

One note: For younger women, quitting may be easier right after the menstrual period is over. Many withdrawal symptoms (anxiety, irritability, weight gain, decreased concentration) *can also be symptoms of Premenstrual Syndrome (PMS)*, and adding additional stress to the premenstrual period may trigger a relapse.

MORE TRIED-AND-TRUE SMOKELESS "URGE TAMERS"

Women in the Smokeless program say the following tips were especially helpful:

Smokeless Inhalation: Every time you feel the urge to smoke, try this: Breathe deeply through the mouth, then hold the breath for three seconds and finally, slowly exhale through pursed lips to make a whispering sound. Do this as many times as you need to until the urge goes away.

Positive Rewards: Save the money you spent weekly on cigarettes and buy yourself little rewards, like a manicure. One woman saved up the money she would have spent on smoking for two months and hired someone to clean her apartment, something she had once thought an impossible luxury.

Eating Management: Drink up to eight glasses of sugar-free liquids a day, both as an appetite suppressant and as a substitute behavior for smoking. Eat regular meals and have plenty of low-calorie snacks on hand. Anything that goes into your mouth instead of a cigarette should be no-cal or low-cal. When dining out, always sit in the no-smoking section.

Smokeless Satisfiers: Chew or suck on sugarless gum or candy, sugar-free breath mints, toothpicks, coffee stirrers, cocktail swizzlers—whatever works for you.

Positive Thinking: Don't think you're "giving up" cigarettes. Instead, believe you're "getting rid of" cigarettes, just like you get rid of the household trash. When you're tempted to smoke, say to yourself: "The urge to smoke will pass, whether or not I light up." Remember: Smoking a cigarette to relieve an urge only creates another urge to smoke. One woman found it helped to say "Stop!" every time she wanted to light up. At first she shouted; now, she just thinks the word.

Don't Get Too "H-A-L-T": Being too Hungry, Anxious, Lonely, or Tired are smoking triggers.

Adapted from Smokeless materials, reprinted by permission of the American Institute for Preventive Medicine, Farmington Hills, Michigan.

Beware of the two biggest reasons for backsliding: stress and being around other smokers, especially in the beginning.

"If you do gain a couple of pounds, don't panic. Once you're feeling comfortable as an ex-smoker, you'll be able to apply those successful behavior-changing strategies to losing weight," says DiFrisco.

Enlist support from friends and family. Warn them that you may be a little hard to live with at first, but you won't appreciate hearing: "You're so irritable, I wish you'd just go back to smoking," says DiFrisco. If family members smoke, ask them to do it out of your presence.

"Keep busy. In the past, if you had ten minutes to kill, you'd probably light up a cigarette. So don't give yourself idle time to slip back into bad habits," counsels DiFrisco.

"If you do give in to an urge to smoke, look at it as a one-time thing, not as a failure. Learn from your mistake and go right back to nonsmoking behavior. Don't let one slip-up become an excuse for giving up. Remember, you *can* kick the habit for good!"

3

Watch Your Blood Pressure

WOMEN MAY PAY a great deal of attention to diet or weight. But many of us forget to keep tabs on blood pressure. That can be a dangerous oversight. Almost 60 percent of deaths attributable to hypertension occur among women.

It's estimated that 27 percent of all women between the ages of eighteen and seventy-four have hypertension. The prevalence goes up to 67.5 percent of women by age sixty-five, and to 72 percent between ages sixty-five and seventy-four. The Framingham Heart Study found that women with high blood pressure have a two to eight times' greater risk of a stroke or heart attack than women with normal blood pressure.

Prevention is important for every woman, and especially vital for those at increased risk: African-American, Latina and Native-American women, as well as women who live in the southeastern United States, the so-called stroke belt.

WHAT IS HIGH BLOOD PRESSURE?

Blood pressure is a measurement of the pressure created against blood vessel walls as blood is pumped from the heart.

The heart beats sixty to seventy times a minute, and with each beat, pumps two or three ounces of oxygen-rich blood through the aorta out to blood vessels all over the body. The pressure from this spurt of blood is called *systolic* blood pressure. That is the higher number in your blood pressure reading.

As the heart rests between beats, blood flows to tissues throughout the body, and the pressure in our blood vessels drops. The pressure during this period is called a resting or *diastolic* blood pressure. This is the lower number in your blood pressure reading.

Blood pressure varies during the day: It's lowest during sleep and highest just before we awaken and when we wake, as the body gets in gear for the day (most heart attacks occur during this vulnerable early morning period). Blood pressure rises during vigorous exercise because our muscles need extra nutrients and oxygen; the heart may beat more than one hundred twenty times a minute, pumping out double or triple the normal amount of blood.

In order to keep up with all this activity, the walls of our blood vessels must expand and contract with each surge of blood. Stiffened or overly constricted arteries resist blood flow. This resistance can cause high blood pressure, since the pressure remains high both when the heart is pumping and at rest.

HOW HYPERTENSION DOES ITS SILENT DAMAGE

The higher your blood pressure, the harder your heart must work to pump blood. Like any muscle forced to work under increased pressure for a long period of time, the heart muscle starts to thicken. But unlike other muscles that work better with extra use, when the heart enlarges, it may become weaker and may not be able to meet the demands put on it. The left ventricle, the heart's main pumping chamber, is the part of the heart muscle most often enlarged by chronic hypertension. The result of this *left ventricular hypertrophy* is congestive heart failure.

In congestive heart failure, the heart fails to deliver enough blood to the kidneys, so the kidneys can't effectively excrete salt and water. Fluid accumulates in body tissues, causing swelling or *edema*, especially in the legs and feet. The lungs may also become waterlogged, making breathing more difficult.

Untreated hypertension also scars and hardens the walls of blood vessels, from the aorta down to the tiniest arterioles in the kidney and the brain, increasing resistance to blood flow. The hardening of the arteries, or *arteriosclerosis*, occurs to some degree over the years as we age, but untreated hypertension speeds it up considerably.

The muscles in blood vessel walls thicken, making it hard for blood to pass through. In the kidney, this can result in a backup of waste products and eventually to kidney failure. In the brain, this can compromise blood flow and, some studies suggest, cause atrophy and shrinkage of the brain. In fact, several 1994 studies found that chronic hypertension in elderly people can lead to declines in mental function, especially in short-term memory and attention, over and above those caused by the natural course of aging. The longer a person's blood pressure was elevated, the greater the decline.

Hypertension is a known risk factor for certain types of stroke, causing blisterlike weak spots called *aneurysms* in artery walls. These aneurysms can burst, causing a hemorrhage. A rupture in a blood vessel in the brain can result in a stroke or even death; a rupture in the aorta can cause a fatal hemorrhage.

Constantly elevated pressure can also cause tiny cracks in the lining of blood vessels. Excess cholesterol may seep underneath and narrow blood vessels further. One of the forms of blood cells that trigger clotting, called *platelets*, can accumulate in these damaged sites and cause a heart attack.

The cells lining the walls of blood vessels, called the *endothelium*, secrete small amounts of a chemical that helps relax blood vessel walls in response to stress. Scientists now know that this mysterious substance is nitric oxide. Nitric oxide is produced in smaller amounts in diseased arteries and seems to be less effective.

High blood pressure can even cause small hemorrhages in the retina, the light-sensitive membrane in the back of the eye, resulting in peripheral or central vision loss.

What's especially insidious about this whole process is that it's so gradual. You may have no symptoms at all until your blood pressure reaches the danger zone and causes a heart attack or stroke. High blood pressure is not called "the silent killer" for nothing.

WHAT THE NUMBERS MEAN TO YOU

The instrument traditionally used to measure blood pressure is called a *sphygmomanometer* (pronounced SFIG-mo-mah-NOM-eh-tur). It consists of an inflatable cuff, an air pump, and a column of mercury in a glass gauge. The two numbers in the blood pressure reading are taken from this gauge in millimeters of mercury, abbreviated as *mmHg*. (Physicians may also use a digital instrument to measure blood pressure.)

The test takes a few moments and should be done in a quiet setting. The cuff is wrapped around your bare arm, and a rubber bulb is used to pump air into the cuff. The cuff is pumped up until it compresses the major artery of the arm and stops blood flow temporarily.

While the cuff is being inflated, the doctor puts a stethoscope in the crook of your elbow to listen to the pulse of blood flow as it decreases, then stops. The air is gradually let out of the cuff and the doctor listens for a thumping sound, which indicates blood is spurting back into the artery. The level or millimeters of mercury when that first thump is heard is the *systolic* or pumping pressure.

As the cuff deflates further, the artery opens more fully; sounds heard through the stethoscope gradually fade. The level of the mercury on the gauge when this happens indicates resting or *diastolic* blood pressure.

A healthy, premenopausal woman can have a blood pressure reading anywhere between 110 mmHg systolic/65 mmHg diastolic to 120 mmHg systolic/80 mmHg diastolic. After menopause, the average blood pressure tends to be slightly higher; between 120/80 to 140/90.

Experts generally agree that "hypertension" is a reading of 140/90 mmHg or higher, confirmed by two consecutive visits to the doctor. But there are shades of difference in the diagnosis.

In 1992, the National High Blood Pressure Education Program lowered the threshold for "normal" blood pressure and replaced the categories of "mild," "moderate" and "severe" hypertension with numerical classifications, in stages one through four.

BLOOD PRESSURE GUIDELINES

CLASSIFICATION	SYSTOLIC (in mmHg)	DIASTOLIC (in mmHg)
Normal	< 130	< 85
High–Normal	130–139	85–99
Stage 1 (formerly Mild)	140–159	90–99
Stage 2 (formerly Moderate)	160–179	100–190
Stage 3 (formerly Severe)	180–209	110–119
Stage 4 (formerly Very Severe)	> 210	> 120

Source: National High Blood Pressure Education Program/National Heart, Lung and Blood Institute, Fifth Joint National Committee Report, 1992.

"The descriptive terms were dropped because the word 'mild' could make people too complacent about controlling their blood pressure," explains Marvin Moser, M.D., a professor of medicine at Yale University and a member of the national committee that drafted the guidelines. "This is especially important, since new evidence shows that some complications can begin when hypertension is in its earliest stages."

A 1993 study found that up to one third of men and women with mildly elevated blood pressure (a diastolic reading between 90 and 99) already showed signs of left ventricular hypertrophy. The condition was more common in smokers, people who were overweight, and ate a diet high in salt.

Having "high normal" blood pressure doesn't necessarily mean you're in any imminent danger of a heart attack or stroke, but your blood pressure does bear watching, stresses Dr. Moser. "If your [systolic] pressure reading is between 130 and 139 and [diastolic] 85 to 89, it does need to be rechecked within a year." Lifestyle changes like losing weight, a lower salt diet and regular exercise will probably be recommended, he adds.

Some people may get a higher blood pressure reading simply because of anxiety at being in the doctor's office. This is aptly called "white coat" hypertension. So repeated measurements may be needed to see if you really do have elevated blood pressure.

MEASURING BLOOD PRESSURE PROPERLY

The National High Blood Pressure Education Program (NHBEP) says a blood pressure exam should begin only after a patient has been resting for at least five minutes and should include two or more readings done at least two minutes apart, averaging the results. If there's a difference of more than five millimeters, additional readings are needed.

Your physician may also take pressure readings while you're lying down, sitting or standing up and may take readings from both arms. People may have a higher reading in one arm, due to arterial blockages affecting one side of the body. To help ensure the accuracy of your test, do not smoke or have any caffeine within thirty minutes of the exam.

Some physicians are now using twenty-four-hour continuous blood pressure monitoring for diagnosis and monitoring the effects of treatment; the NHBEP does not recommend ambulatory monitoring as a routine test. It is expensive and advised only for patients who need evaluation of possible resistance to antihypertensive medication and those experiencing symptoms associated with medication. Home blood pressure monitoring with an inexpensive device may give just as much information, Dr. Moser adds.

WHAT MAY CAUSE
BLOOD PRESSURE TO RISE

Between 90 and 95 percent of all cases of adult high blood pressure are classified *essential* or *primary hypertension*, for which there is no one underlying cause.

About 5 percent of all cases of high blood pressure are caused by disease, such as kidney disorders. This is called *secondary hypertension*, and treating the cause will usually help control this form of hypertension. Recent research suggests these other culprits elevate blood pressure:

Smoking: Each cigarette you smoke may raise your blood pressure by as much as twenty points. Some experts believe that long-term smoking may lead to hypertension due to the constant constriction of blood vessels caused by the chemicals in cigarette smoke. Smoking may also affect certain adrenal hormones that control salt and water metabolism. When the body retains too much fluid, plasma volume increases and blood pressure rises.

Stimulants: Alcohol can cause constriction of blood vessels and, over time, may contribute to hypertension. A recent Boston University study of more than three thousand men and women found drinking more than three ounces of alcohol a week raised the risk of high blood pressure; the more alcohol consumed, the higher the risk. Alcohol may also interfere with antihypertensive medications.

Cocaine, crack cocaine and amphetamines cause the body to produce excess stress hormones, which severely constricts arteries, drastically raises heart rate and boosts blood pressure.

High-Salt Diet: In about half of all people with high blood pressure (the percentage is even higher among African Americans), high salt intake may contribute to hypertension. Salt helps regulate the body's fluid balance. In so-called salt-sensitive people, the kidneys are unable to excrete excess salt. Water and sodium accumulate in the tissues, and the heart has to work harder to pump blood to swollen tissues; blood plasma levels also rise, and the result is high blood pressure.

Mineral Deficiencies: According to the latest research, too little calcium in the diet may trigger high blood pressure in some salt-sensitive people. Calcium is normally needed by muscle cells to contract. It's theorized that when salt-sensitive people eat too much sodium, it sends a hormonal signal to the muscle cells in blood vessels to let in *extra* calcium, causing them to overconstrict. If a salt-sensitive person gets enough calcium, this hormonal signal is blocked and blood vessels won't overconstrict.

Since many people—particularly African Americans and Native Americans—are lactose intolerant (they cannot digest milk sugar), they avoid dairy products, and this could be a factor in the increased risk of hypertension among those groups.

Magnesium and potassium also play a role in regulating blood pressure. Magnesium may help blood vessels relax, and so a deficiency may cause overconstriction. It's theorized that potassium may block absorption of sodium by the kidneys or may help them get rid of excess salt and water, lowering blood plasma volume. So getting too little potassium could also contribute to fluid retention.

Mounting evidence supports these theories, including a report from the Nurses' Health Study which found women whose diets were low in calcium and magnesium had a 23 percent greater chance of developing high blood pressure. In addition, the National Health and Nutrition Examination Survey (NHANES) found that people who consumed less than 1,200 milligrams of potassium a day had two times the incidence of hypertension as people who consumed over 3,600 milligrams a day.

While experts caution more data are needed to confirm these findings, many scientists are beginning to look at calcium, magnesium and potassium supplements as a way of controlling some cases of hypertension (see pages 112–116).

Obesity: Being more than 20 percent over an ideal body weight can increase the resistance to blood flow in smaller blood vessels. People who are obese also tend to become insulin resistant, which may lead to diabetes and often to hypertension as well. The Framingham Heart Study found overweight people are eight times more likely to become diabetic than thinner people. Obesity is more prevalent among African-American and Native-American women, two groups at especially high risk for hypertension.

Diabetes: Diabetes occurs when the body does not produce or respond normally to insulin, the hormone that helps the body break down carbohydrates (particularly sugars) so that they can be used for energy. When there's not enough insulin, too much sugar remains in the blood and can damage the heart, blood vessels and kidneys. Nerve damage may also mute the pain of ischemia.

There are two main types of diabetes: *Type I, juvenile or insulin-dependent diabetes;* and *Type II, noninsulin-dependent diabetes.* Pregnant women may also develop a temporary form of diabetes called *gestational diabetes.*

In Type I diabetes, the cells that produce insulin in the pancreas are damaged or destroyed by the body's own immune system. The process that triggers this destruction is not fully understood. (New research suggests the trigger may be a virus.) It can come on suddenly, usually before age twenty. People with Type I diabetes must receive injected insulin in order to survive.

In Type II diabetes, a person becomes "resistant" to insulin. That is, the body is not able to effectively use the insulin it makes. This process starts gradually, usually in people who are over age forty and overweight.

In a premenopausal woman, diabetes cancels out estrogen's protective effects.

Of all cases of diabetes, 90 percent are Type II and can be controlled through weight loss, diet and exercise (measures that also help control high blood pressure). Type II diabetes is more common in women than men, and more prevalent among black, Native-American and Latina women than among white women.

Race and Hypertension: African Americans in general run twice the risk of hypertension as that of whites. Black women are at *especially* great risk of hypertension, even very young black women, because many have more than one risk factor, including obesity and Type II diabetes, as well as a possible genetic tendency for blood pressure to rise when they eat too much salt.

Data released at a 1994 American Heart Association conference on heart disease in African-American women revealed that high blood pressure is 1.7 times more common in black women than in whites. Between ages sixty-five to seventy-three, the prevalence of high blood pressure among black women is 73 percent, compared to 53 percent of whites. Hypertension also develops earlier, is undertreated and has more severe complications in black women.

Almost 44 percent of all African-American women are overweight, compared to one quarter of white women. The rate of diabetes is as much as 50 percent higher among African-American women, compared to whites, with obesity being a major contributing factor. Death rates for hypertension among black women are about five times higher than among white women.

Research presented at a 1994 conference on hypertension in blacks suggests that African Americans may have less flexible blood vessels than whites.

Some experts suggest that socioeconomic factors may play a role. One study from Johns Hopkins posits that the stress of poverty and racism may induce a hormonal response that constricts arteries and sends blood pressure soaring in African Americans. Another study, from the University of Maryland at College Park, found blood vessels in blacks given a stress test stayed constricted ten times longer than those of whites because of a hormone associated with the skin pigment melanin.

It was also recently reported that people who lack a regular doctor (a common situation among many inner-city blacks) were more likely to have severe high blood pressure that needed emergency treatment than those who have a primary care physician. The high cost of medical care and lack of medical insurance may also prevent low-income patients from getting screened and treated for hypertension.

GENES, HYPERTENSION AND AFRICAN AMERICANS

Clarence E. Grim, M.D., director of the Drew/UCLA Hypertension Research Center at the Charles R. Drew University of Medicine and Science in Los Angeles, theorizes that African Americans' inherited tendency to retain salt (which makes them more prone to salt-sensitive hypertension) is a trait that evolved due to the many deaths from starvation, salt loss and dehydration during the days of slave ships. Those Africans who could retain salt—and, therefore, water—survived the journey to the New World and could endure the ensuing conditions of slavery (as could their descendents).

But Dr. Grim says the salt-retaining gene today makes present-day African Americans sensitive to the effects of sodium in their diet. To prove their point, Dr. Grim and his team of researchers traveled to rural Nigeria. They found that while blacks in both countries ate a diet high in salt, only African Americans had hypertension (most likely of the "salt-sensitive" type). In addition, DNA analyses of blacks in Barbados indicated that those with a maternal African heritage had higher-than-normal blood pressure than those who had no maternal genetic links to Africa.

Although no one has yet found an actual salt-retaining gene, Dr. Grim's research team did find a possible genetic marker that could one day lead to a test that might help predict which African Americans are more susceptible to high blood pressure.

Other theories about hereditary hypertension and blacks involve the enzymes *aldosterone* and *renin*. Aldosterone is secreted by the adrenal gland and helps the kidneys regulate sodium and water balance in the body; overproduction causes salt and water retention. Renin is produced by the kidneys and, when released into the blood, activates another hormone called *angiotensin* to constrict blood vessels. Dr. Grim notes that African Americans have a greater prevalence of hypertension associated with high aldosterone and low renin.

Dr. Grim's take-home message for African-American women: Remember your history and its consequences—a tendency to retain salt. And while this research is still very preliminary, it would probably be wise for women to lower their salt intake (and their family's) to well below 2,000 milligrams a day, add more calcium and potassium-rich foods to their diets and keep their weight down (as well as their children's weights). Avoiding high-salt, high-fat fast-foods and learning how to prepare favorite dishes without a lot of salt may also go a long way in preventing high blood pressure among blacks.

Genetics: Experts have long known that having a parent who has high blood pressure greatly increased a person's chances of developing the disease. Recent reports have identified a number of genes that may lead to hypertension and high blood pressure during pregnancy.

Advancing Age: Before menopause, women generally have lower blood pressures than men of the same age. Between the ages of fifty-five and sixty-five, however, women and men share the same risk of getting high blood pressure. After age sixty-five, women are twice as likely as men to develop high blood pressure. Some experts suggest the cessation of estrogen production may reduce blood vessel dilation (see Chapter 10).

About three million Americans over age sixty have a condition called *isolated systolic hypertension,* or *ISH.* ISH occurs when blood pressure is elevated while the heart beats, but is normal while the heart rests. ISH is thought to be caused by loss of elasticity in the aorta due to arteriosclerosis, and is more common in women than men; ISH affects as many as two thirds of women ages sixty-five to eighty-nine.

HIGH BLOOD PRESSURE AND PREGNANCY

When a woman is pregnant, every organ works harder, including the heart and kidneys. Blood volume increases by nearly 50 percent to supply both the mother and fetus with oxygen and vital nutrients. To help the circulatory system accommodate this increased blood volume, two body chemicals called *prostaglandins* help blood vessels expand and contract as needed. One, *thromboxane,* causes blood vessels to constrict while the other, *prostacyclin,* helps blood vessels relax. When the delicate balance of these two chemicals is upset, a temporary pregnancy-induced hypertension results.

It's estimated that up to 12 percent of all pregnancies are complicated by hypertensive disorders; the majority of these women have a potentially serious condition called *preeclampsia* or *toxemia*.

Preeclampsia/Toxemia: The actual cause of preeclampsia is not known. It usually develops after the midpoint in pregnancy, at about twenty weeks, when the mother's blood volume reaches its peak. Preeclampsia is most common in first-time pregnancies, women over age thirty-five, diabetics, as well as women who are overweight or carrying more than one fetus. Women who have more than one child and who have previously existing hypertension are at a 25 percent greater risk of developing preeclampsia.

When a woman's blood flow is restricted due to hypertension, the fetus may become malnourished and oxygen-starved. Preeclampsia is implicated in one quarter of premature deliveries in the United States and can increase the risk of a low-birthweight baby and stillbirth. In extreme cases, weakened blood vessels leading to the placenta may cause the placenta to tear away from the uterine wall (*abruptio placentae*), leading to hemorrhage and premature birth.

Pregnant women get routine high blood pressure and urine checks, but women should also be extra alert for the physical symptoms during their pregnancy.

PREECLAMPSIA WARNING SIGNS

Alert your doctor if you experience *any* of these symptoms:

- Sudden weight gain of over two pounds a week
- Swelling in the hands, legs, feet or face
- A headache that won't go away
- Dizziness or blurred vision

Pregnant women are also advised to decrease their salt intake and get more calcium. A recent report in the *New England Journal of Medicine* suggests that taking two grams of calcium a day, starting in twentieth week of pregnancy might help prevent preeclampsia. If a woman is overweight, she should try to get her weight down to normal levels before becoming pregnant.

If preeclampsia is left untreated, it can progress to a more severe stage called maternal eclampsia, which can lead to convulsions, organ failure, coma and even death. But most cases of preeclampsia are caught early and are treated with a combination of bed rest and antihypertensive drugs.

A woman with preeclampsia may be advised to lie on her left side several times a day to improve circulation to her uterus and other organs, since blood exits the heart from the left side and lying on the left helps this along.

Transient hypertension may occur at any time or in the first twenty-four hours after delivery, without other signs of preeclampsia or preexisting hypertension. Transient hypertension puts a woman at risk of developing hypertension later in life.

This condition is treated in much the same way as high blood pressure in nonpregnant women. However, a class of drugs called *ACE inhibitors* (see page 51) may cause injury to a fetus.

ASPIRIN AND PREECLAMPSIA

A number of recent studies suggest that *small* daily doses of aspirin may reduce the risk of pregnancy-induced hypertension for women at high risk of preeclampsia. Experts believe that aspirin inhibits production of the prostaglandin thromboxane, which causes blood-vessel constriction.

An analysis of six clinical trials shows 65 percent of women at *high risk* for preeclampsia who took *low* daily doses of aspirin (60–150 mg) in the last two trimesters of pregnancy reduced their risk of toxemia, compared with women who did not take aspirin.

One randomized, controlled clinical trial involving 3,135 women expecting their first child and who had *normal blood pressure* found those women who took sixty milligrams of aspirin a day had a 26 percent lower incidence of preeclampsia compared with women taking a placebo. However, the risk reduction was mainly confined to those women whose initial systolic pressure was slightly elevated (120–134 mmHg). The trial, reported in 1993 in the *New England Journal of Medicine*, also found that taking aspirin slightly increased the risk of abruptio placentae.

The authors of the study recommend that aspirin *not* be used as a prophylactic in first-time pregnancies in healthy women. Aspirin interferes with blood clotting and could increase the chances of maternal bleeding, especially when taken up to five days before delivery. Aspirin may also have some damaging effects to the fetus's cardiovascular system, causing premature closure of a vital blood vessel, which could lead to heart failure.

Bottom line: Do *not* take aspirin during pregnancy unless your doctor prescribes it.

BLOOD PRESSURE AND THE PILL

Women who have high blood pressure or other vascular problems should *not* take oral contraceptives, because it can increase their risk of stroke. There is also a very slight risk of developing hypertension on the pill; higher doses of the synthetic estrogen and progesterone in the pill may increase blood volume and increased resistance in small blood vessels.

Women who smoke and take birth control pills run a 40 percent higher relative risk of developing cardiovascular disease, specially strokes. This is true even for today's low-dose pills. If a physician detects a blood pressure problem, discontinuing the pill should bring pressure back to normal.

If you are taking oral contraceptives, you need to see your doctor every six months for checks of blood pressure and cholesterol levels. (For more on the pill, see Chapter 9.)

LOWERING YOUR BLOOD PRESSURE

If you have high blood pressure, simple lifestyle changes may help. These include quitting smoking if you're a smoker, losing weight if you're overweight, a low-salt diet (for those who are salt-sensitive), reducing alcohol intake and a program of regular exercise.

Sodium intake should be less than six grams a day. Since alcohol can raise blood pressure, new federal guidelines call for limiting daily alcohol intake to two ounces of 100-proof whiskey, eight ounces of wine or twenty-four ounces of beer.

These kinds of lifestyle changes may help 15 to 25 percent of people lower high blood pressure.

Exercise can have a potent effect on blood pressure. Recent studies in the United States and England found that for some people with mild to moderate hypertension, aerobic exercise—such as brisk walking for thirty minutes a day at least three times a week—may be effective all by itself in lowering blood pressure. One reason, of course, is that exercise promotes weight loss, which alone helps lower blood pressure. People who exercise regularly also tend to have lower pulse rates.

Researchers at Harvard say that for every one point reduction in elevated diastolic blood pressure, a woman reduces her risk of heart attack by 2 to 3 percent. Based on the results of typical treatment, a woman could cut her heart attack risk by up to 20 percent by diet and exercise alone.

DRUGS THAT LOWER BLOOD PRESSURE

If three to six months of rigorous lifestyle changes fail to lower blood pressure sufficiently, new treatment guidelines from the National High Blood Pressure Education Program suggest that patients begin drug therapy (see pages 50–52).

Four important recent randomized clinical trials show that drug therapy can benefit women with high blood pressure:

• The Treatment of Mild Hypertension Study (TOMHS) found that in men and women with mild (Stage I) hypertension, treatment with a combination of drug therapy and lifestyle changes reduced heart attacks and stroke in men and women by 32 percent.

• The Systolic Hypertension in the Elderly Program (SHEP) trial found that treating isolated systolic hypertension in women over age sixty with a low dose of diuretic (chlorthalidone) cut the risk of heart disease and stroke by about one third.

• The Medical Research Council Trial (MRCT) in Great Britain, involving men and women between ages sixty-five and seventy-four (43 percent of whom had ISH), found diuretics were more effective than beta blockers in women in reducing hypertension.

• A three-year Swedish trial which involved about eight hundred people ages seventy to eighty-four with high blood pressure (almost two thirds of whom were women) found treatment with diuretics or beta blockers significantly reduced strokes and deaths from other causes.

At the same time, other recent research has raised questions about the side effects and effectiveness of antihypertensive treatments in women. Certain diuretics and beta blockers may raise women's total blood cholesterol and LDL, while lowering levels of the "good" HDL cholesterol; recent studies with diuretics indicate if changes do occur, they may disappear within a year. Antihypertensive medications may cause sexual dysfunction in women as well as in men. In addition, recent research suggests that some drug treatments may not be as effective in white women under age sixty-five as they are in black women.

There is also new evidence that hormone replacement therapy after menopause may slightly help in controlling blood pressure. But the research is extremely preliminary (see Chapter 10).

Different medications may be more suitable for women in certain situations, such as during pregnancy, after age sixty, or if a woman has diabetes or osteoporosis. Older women may require smaller doses of medication, since the body gets rid of drugs more slowly as we age. The NHPEP recommends the initial dose of medication for an elderly person should be half that prescribed for younger patients.

New treatment guidelines suggest that diuretics first be prescribed by themselves, or in combination with beta blockers for the treatment of hypertension. Diuretics and newer drugs like calcium channel blockers may be especially effective in African Americans.

Experts say the major problem is getting people to *stay* on medications. Since hypertension often has no symptoms until there's a heart attack or stroke, it's often difficult to convince people that they really need medication when they don't feel ill. Some people quit taking medication and may stop seeing their doctor. The result: Their blood pressure rises again and they may never know. So if your doctor prescribes a medication, don't stop taking it for any reason, or take it less often, unless he or she instructs you to.

One thing to know: Drug therapy isn't always forever. In some patients, when a combination of lifestyle changes and medications lowers blood pressure, it's possible to reduce doses or (in some cases) even eliminate medication if other nondrug regimens are continued and the patient is carefully monitored.

A 1994 study found that mildly obese people (either taking a single blood pressure drug or no medication) are more likely to remain off additional drug therapy if they follow a weight-loss program and a low-sodium/high-potassium diet.

BLOOD PRESSURE MEDICATIONS

Diuretics: Diuretics help the kidney get rid of excess salt and fluid, reducing blood volume, which lightens the load on the heart. Diuretics also help blood vessels to relax. Diuretics are especially effective for people with salt-sensitive hypertension.

There are three different types of diuretics:

• Thiazide diuretics such as chlorthacidone (Hygroton) work in the network of distal tubules in the kidney, which transport urine.

• Loop diuretics, including furosemide (Lasix) get their name because they work in an area of the kidney called the "loop of Henle." They are less commonly used, since they cause more fluid loss and other side effects.

• Potassium-sparing diuretics, such as amiloride (Midamor), affect the area of the kidney where potassium is excreted. They prevent excessive loss of potassium; low doses are often used in conjunction with the two other types of diuretics.

Potential Side Effects: In low doses, diuretics have minimal side effects, if any. However, some studies have shown that higher doses of these drugs can increase cholesterol and blood sugar temporarily and may flush too much potassium from the body along with excess salt and water. In very rare cases, diuretics can cause stomach irritations or ulcers. They can also interact with other medications, including aspirinlike drugs. Other side effects can include dizziness, electrolyte imbalances, muscle cramps, nausea, joint pain, hearing loss and sexual dysfunction. One study found that thiazide diuretics may protect against hip fracture in older women.

Warning: Those taking diuretics need to have their cholesterol, blood sugar and potassium levels checked periodically. Dizziness or muscle cramps may be a sign of electrolyte imbalance and should be reported to a physician.

Beta Blockers: These medications, including propranolol (Inderal), metoprolol (Lopressor) and labetalol (Normodyne), block the effects of chemicals produced by the sympathetic nervous system, decreasing cardiac contractions and slowing the heart rate.

Because they slow heart rate, these drugs work particularly well in patients who have angina or who have had a prior heart attack. Beta blockers can also reduce anxiety in some patients.

Potential Side Effects: Beta blockers have side effects including sluggishness and depression; some women report they have difficulty achieving orgasm (some men suffer impotence). In some cases, beta blockers may worsen asthma, congestive heart failure, and other conditions. They can also interact with anticlotting and cholesterol-lowering drugs.

Warning: In very rare instances, beta blockers can impair electrical rhythms in the heart, causing "heart block." Doses of beta blockers need to be carefully regulated, and those taking these drugs must be monitored by their physician.

ACE Inhibitors: ACE stands for *angiotensin-converting enzyme*, which raises blood pressure by constricting the smooth muscle cells in blood vessel walls. ACE inhibitors, like enalapril (Vaseretic) or captopril (Capozide), interfere with the action of the enzyme, vasoconstriction. ACE inhibitors also lower blood pressure by interfering with renin's effects.

Potential Side Effects: The most common effect (in about 15 percent of people) is a cough. Other side effects may include weakness and allergic reactions ranging from swelling to skin rashes; ACE inhibitors can also worsen kidney disease.

Warning: ACE inhibitors are not recommended for use during pregnancy; they may cause injury or death to a fetus when given during the second or third trimester. Exposure during the first trimester does not appear to have adverse effects, but a woman taking ACE inhibitors who becomes pregnant should contact her physician, since alternate medication is needed.

Calcium Channel Blockers: All muscles, including those in the heart and blood vessels, need calcium to contract. In some hypertensives, extra calcium is thought to be sent into blood vessels, which contract and raise blood pressure. Calcium channel blockers, like diltiazem (Cardizem), nifedipine (Procardia) and verapamil (Calan), prevent this from happening.

Potential Side Effects: These drugs seem to be very effective with fewer side effects than some beta blockers.

Warning: They may worsen congestive heart failure and, like beta blockers, cause heart block, so they're not for every patient.

Vasodilators: Like hydralazine (Apresoline) and minoxidil (Loniten) (yes, the same chemical being used topically to treat hair loss), vasodilators act directly on blood vessel walls to prevent constriction or stimulate dilation. These are potent medications used when other drugs aren't effective. Minoxidil is given with diuretics and sometimes beta blockers.
  Potential Side Effects: Common side effects can include dizziness, nausea, vomiting, headaches and irregular heartbeats. Minoxidil can increase hair growth, cause rashes, headaches, fluid retention and shortness of breath. Consult a physician before using over-the-counter cold remedies and ibuprofen.

Aplha Blockers: These drugs block nerve receptors known as alpha receptors in the autonomic nervous system which normally help constrict the arterioles. Alpha blockers lower blood pressure and reduce the work load of the heart in people suffering from heart failure. These drugs, including prazosin (Minipress), and doxazosin (Cardura), also reduce the action of the stress hormone norepinephrine. They are usually given with other blood pressure drugs such as diuretics or beta blockers.
  Potential Side Effects: Side effects may include a drop in blood pressure when a person moves from a sitting or prone position to standing, resulting in dizziness or a fainting spell. Diuretics increase the blood-pressure-lowering ability of some alpha blockers. Alpha blockers may also cause headaches, palpitations and nausea.

Central Alpha Agonists: These drugs stimulate brain centers to lessen nerve impulses that cause blood vessels to constrict. Central alpha agonists like methyldopa (Aldomet), clonidine (Catapres) and guanabenz (Wytensin) are not often used as first-line medications for hypertension. They may be given in combination with other drugs if other therapy fails.
  Potential Side Effects: Side effects may include drowsiness, headache, dry mouth, constipation, swelling of ankles or feet, depression and, in the case of methyldopa, liver inflammation.

Sources: *Physicians' Desk Reference, 1993; United States Pharmacopeia 1993, Complete Drug Reference; Consumer Reports* books; National High Blood Pressure Education Program/NHLBI, *Fifth Joint National Committee Report, 1992.*

DIET: BEYOND THE SALTSHAKER

For years, the conventional wisdom was that a low-salt diet could reduce your risk of high blood pressure. The fact is, only about half of people with high blood pressure are "sensitive" to sodium. However, as many as 80 percent of African Americans with hypertension may be in this group.

Short-term trials show that moderate sodium restriction can reduce systolic blood pressure by almost 5 millimeters and diastolic pressure by 2.6 millimeters. Blood pressure is reduced even further if salt is restricted over the long term.

In addition, since calcium deficiencies can make salt-sensitive hypertension worse, it's important to get enough calcium in the diet. Magnesium is also needed to maintain elasticity of blood vessels, and potassium helps the body regulate the balance of salt and water; deficiencies may cause high blood pressure.

Federal experts are not yet recommending mineral supplements for lowering high blood pressure. But recent studies suggest they may help:

• Researchers at the Oregon Health Sciences University found that people with mild hypertension who took a one-gram calcium supplement each day for eight weeks lowered their blood pressure to normal ranges. Among African Americans who had a low calcium intake, another study found calcium supplements significantly lowered blood pressure.

• An Italian study cited in the *Annals of Internal Medicine* found that people with high blood pressure who ate a diet high in potassium were able to control their blood pressure with half the usual amount of medication.

• A report from the University of California at Los Angeles suggests magnesium supplements may also help lower blood pressure in people with noninsulin-dependent diabetes.

The blood pressure reductions in some of these studies were fairly modest. But for people with borderline hypertension, that may be enough to bring pressure down to normal levels.

In the meantime, experts recommend that people have at least the minimum daily allowance of 800–1,500 milligrams of calcium (in food or calcium supplements). Since many African Americans are lactose intolerant, calcium supplements might be a good idea, along with eating more fruits and vegetables (like greens) rich in calcium.

Scientists also recommend at least 400 milligrams a day of magnesium and 1,600–2,000 milligrams of potassium, which can be easily obtained through diet. Just one banana has 400 milligrams of potassium. (For details on food high in calcium, magnesium and potassium, see Chapter 6.)

By the way, one food that may *raise* blood pressure, if eaten in excess, is real black licorice. A chemical in licorice (not in licorice flavoring), called *glycyrrhizinic acid*, is known to constrict blood vessels.

AN OUNCE OF PREVENTION

There *are* proven steps you can take to *prevent* hypertension. The National High Blood Pressure Education Program's new prevention guidelines are as follows:

• Consume no more than one teaspoon of table salt, or 2,400 milligrams of sodium, a day.

• Lose weight if you are overweight. About 20 to 30 percent of hypertension is related to excess weight.

• Exercise regularly (at least thirty minutes a day, three to five times a week, of moderate aerobic exercise).

• Limit daily alcohol intake to no more than two drinks daily (that's twenty-four ounces of beer, eight ounces of wine and two ounces of 100-proof whiskey).

• Diet should include the recommended daily amounts of calcium, magnesium and potassium.

Along with reducing stress, quitting smoking and cutting fat intake, following these five rules should help protect most women from other cardiovascular diseases, including stroke and atherosclerosis.

4

Cut Back Fat
and Cholesterol

OVER THE PAST twenty years, the cholesterol levels of Americans have taken a decided drop. Even so, more than half of all adult women in this country still have blood cholesterol levels above the level considered healthy.

Having high cholesterol in addition to other cardiac risk factors can substantially increase a woman's chance of having a heart attack. But making changes in your diet and starting an exercise program are often all that's needed to bring down high cholesterol—and lower your heart-disease risk.

HOW DO YOU GET HIGH CHOLESTEROL?

Cholesterol itself is *not* harmful. It's a natural, fatty substance produced by the liver (and to a lesser extent by other cells in the body). Cholesterol is needed to make cell membranes, protective coatings for nerves, to form bile acids used to help digest foods and to provide raw material for sex hormones, including estrogen.

Cholesterol only becomes a problem when the body produces more cholesterol than it needs or can process; the excess circulates in the bloodstream and can contribute to clogging of coronary arteries, explains William Castelli, M.D., director of the Framingham Heart Study.

Just as oil and water don't mix, fat doesn't dissolve in blood plasma (which is mostly water). Fat molecules, or *lipids*, have to be transported through the blood by carriers called *lipoproteins*, fat-filled molecules with a special coating that allows them to dissolve in blood. There are several types of lipoproteins, and they work in different ways.

The two major cholesterol carriers in the blood are *low-density lipoproteins*, or *LDL*, the so-called "bad" cholesterol, and *high-density lipoproteins*, or *HDL*, the "good" cholesterol. LDL carries most of our cholesterol; it not only delivers cholesterol to body tissues, but can also deposit it on artery walls. HDL helps the body get rid of unneeded cholesterol.

Another type of blood fat that can be harmful in excess is *triglycerides*, or *TGL* for short. TGL is produced from carbohydrates and fats in food and is either used for energy by our muscles or stored in fatty tissues.

When we eat fat and cholesterol, the intestines pack them into molecules called *chylomicrons*, which are easily carried by the blood to the liver. The liver then repackages them into *very low-density lipoproteins*, or *VLDL*, and sends them out to the body. As cells remove triglycerides from VLDL to be used for energy, they shrink and become LDL molecules. LDL molecules are then taken up by cells for membrane production or repair and for making hormones. Other fats are repackaged by the liver as HDL.

When we eat too much saturated fat, the body is forced to make more VLDL in an effort to process the extra fat. We end up with too much LDL in the blood because our cells can't handle the overload. LDL receptors on their surface shut down and simply won't let any more inside, says Dr. Castelli. A recent report suggests that hypercholesteremia in women is mainly due to reduced activity of LDL receptors; it's believed that estrogen may increase the number of active LDL receptors in the liver.

Scientists now know that excess LDL can react with oxygen in the body and become *oxidized*, or rancid. Oxidized LDL is taken into scavenger cells called *macrophages*, which help rid the body of unwanted substances. These macrophages become so inflated with fat that they look bubbly, so they're often called foam cells. When the inner lining of the arteries becomes damaged, these cholesterol-loaded foam cells get inside and attract more foam cells, forming a deposit called *plaque*.

This can become a vicious cycle, as more foam cells are drawn in from the blood and more LDL is oxidized. (It's believed that "antioxidant" nutrients, like vitamin E, may help prevent this process. See page 109.)

When fatty plaques get too thick, the opening (or *lumen*) of the arteries supplying the heart can become so narrowed that blood flow is slowed down or blocked. In addition, plaques can rupture. The body's attempt to heal the lesion in the artery attracts immune cells and platelets in the blood, which form clots.

Most heart attacks are caused by a blood clot plugging up an already narrowed coronary artery. When blood is cut off from the heart, the heart muscle starts to die from lack of oxygen. If enough heart muscle dies, the heart can't work well, or fails. Fatty deposits on blood vessel walls can also interfere with blood flow to the brain, causing a stroke.

One third to one fourth of cholesterol in the blood is carried by high-density lipoproteins. HDL carry unused cholesterol away from the arteries and back to the liver, where it is secreted into bile, sent into the intestines and flushed from the body. Recent research indicates that HDL may also remove cholesterol from atherosclerotic plaques and actually slow their growth.

The amount of HDL in relation to other blood fats is now known to be an important predictor for heart disease. The less HDL you have, the less able the body will be to rid itself of extra cholesterol. The key number here is the ratio of LDL to HDL; if it's over four to one you may be in trouble, says Dr. Castelli.

A 1994 study in the American Heart Association journal *Circulation* found that triglycerides are an artery-clogger all by themselves. The two-year study of 270 people found that even after LDL cholesterol was aggressively lowered by drugs, TGL continued to contribute to the growth of smaller lesions in blood vessels leading to the heart. These small, new lesions may be more dangerous than large ones because they are more likely to rupture and block an artery. High triglycerides may be especially dangerous for women.

There are important gender differences in blood fats between men and women as they age.

Cholesterol in the blood is measured in terms of milligrams per deciliter of blood, abbreviated as *mg/dl.* At birth, our total cholesterol measures about 70 mg/dl. By one year of age, it's up to 150 mg/dl. Cholesterol levels stay the same for healthy boys and girls until puberty.

When women reach puberty, the female hormone estrogen allows them to hang on to their HDL cholesterol a little better than men; their HDL remains around 55 mg/dl until menopause. When boys enter puberty, the surge in the male hormone testosterone triggers a rise in their

LDL levels, apparently to build and repair muscles, while their HDL levels fall to about 45 mg/dl. Rather than building muscle in adolescence, women develop fat stores and breasts. It's theorized that women have extra HDL to help control cholesterol during pregnancy, when other blood fats rise.

When men arrive at middle age, their cholesterol levels start rising dramatically. Perhaps because they're less active, LDL once needed to build muscles may remain in the blood and can end up on coronary artery walls. After menopause, women's cholesterol levels actually surpass those of men, so women end up having heart attacks ten years later than men, possibly sooner if they have a family history of heart disease and high cholesterol.

As both sexes get past age sixty, fats also may be removed from the blood less efficiently, giving cholesterol more time to hang around and promote heart disease. Having diabetes also speeds up the process of atherosclerosis; more than half of people with diabetes also have a lipid abnormality.

That doesn't mean that women's coronary arteries are totally clear before menopause and suddenly become clogged afterward, cautions Dr. Castelli. Just like men, women accumulate fatty plaques; but they may be accumulating them at a slower level.

High cholesterol can, and does, occur at any age. A 1993 report in the *Journal of the American Medical Association* says 20 percent of women ages twenty to thirty-nine may have blood cholesterol levels so high they will need treatment. Between ages forty and fifty-nine, the number rises to 47 percent; between ages sixty and seventy-four, 58 percent of women may need treatment for high cholesterol. However, only 12 percent of all women who need it are actually being treated.

THE OTHER "BAD" CHOLESTEROL

There's another "bad" form of cholesterol that we may need to be concerned about. It's called *lipoprotein a or Lp(a)* and it can be a risk factor for heart attacks and strokes.

Lp(a) is an LDL particle with special protein attached to it. As a cholesterol carrier, Lp(a) can help deposit cholesterol and other debris on artery walls and appears to stimulate overgrowth of the smooth muscle cells within artery walls, thickening and clogging key blood vessels. In addition, high levels of Lp(a) also seem to inhibit the body's natural clot-dissolving mechanism.

Lp(a) may be responsible for 25 percent of heart attacks that occur early in life. One 1994 study found that people with high levels of Lp(a) were twenty times more likely to suffer strokes than people with lower levels.

A person's Lp(a) may be genetically determined and, unlike LDL, is not affected by dietary changes or exercise. Higher Lp(a) levels are more common among African Americans. Lp(a) also rises in some women after menopause, but research suggests estrogen replacement may help lower Lp(a).

Desirable levels of Lp(a) are less than 0.3 grams per liter of blood. High Lp(a) may be especially dangerous when LDL is also high, or other coronary risk factors are present. You can be tested for Lp(a) at some research laboratories and major medical centers. But experts caution that clinical studies haven't yet fully proven the predictive value of Lp(a) testing.

PAT'S STORY

"My grandfather had heart problems and quite a few relatives on both sides of the family have high cholesterol. But when I got my cholesterol checked during my annual physical, I couldn't believe how high mine was: 260. I didn't think you could have cholesterol problems this young. I'm only thirty-nine.

"After that, I started to really think about what I was eating. I had been using a lot of prepackaged foods because there was no time to cook for my husband and myself after work. But when I started reading package labels, I could not believe how much fat was in them! I'm eating more vegetables than I ever did. And I never did like vegetables, even as a kid. I only drink skim milk now.

"I used to go to an aerobics class. But I have a pretty hectic schedule. I just had a baby girl a year ago and I work three days a week. I worry about my weight. I haven't been able to lose as much as I'd like. But I try to ride my bike as much as possible and take the baby for long walks. My LDL has gone down; so have my triglycerides."

HORMONAL PROTECTION CONFIRMED

Several recent studies have confirmed that estrogen *does* help maintain high levels of HDL, the "good" cholesterol, and keep total cholesterol low before menopause—and that it can do so after menopause, if women take replacement estrogen.

A study at the University of Pittsburgh followed changes in LDL and HDL levels in over five hundred women ages forty-two to fifty for over two and a half years. In the group, 101 stopped menstruating and 32 began taking replacement estrogen. Their cholesterol levels were compared with women the same age who had not reached menopause.

According to principal investigator Karen A. Matthews, Ph.D., levels of HDL cholesterol among women in the study group dropped 4 mg/dl after they went through menopause, while their LDL levels rose 12 mg/dl. Women who took estrogen supplements had no changes in cholesterol.

Scientists at the Southwest Foundation for Biomedical Research in San Antonio, Texas, suggest that the hormones estrogen and progesterone *together* protect women from heart disease before menopause. They showed that progesterone, which is still produced in the body after the ovaries stop making estrogen, caused blood cholesterol to rise.

Because of the threat of uterine cancer from giving estrogens alone, most women receive a combination of synthetic estrogen and progesterone. A three-year study was begun in 1989 to determine if adding progesterone in hormone replacement therapy interferes with estrogen's protective effects. Preliminary data from the Post-Menopausal Estrogen and Progestin Intervention (PEPI) Trial indicates that oral estrogen can lower LDL and raise HDL, cutting the risk of heart disease by as much as 25 percent. Adding progestins produced a lesser reduction in HDL, but was still beneficial. (For details on the PEPI Trial, see page 168.)

WHAT THE NUMBERS MEAN TO YOU

There are three basic numbers you need to know: your total blood cholesterol, your level of "good" HDL cholesterol versus "bad" LDL cholesterol, and your level of triglycerides.

Total Cholesterol: The 1993 National Cholesterol Education Program Guidelines classify total cholesterol risk as follows:

Under 200 mg/dl	=	Desirable Blood Cholesterol
200–239 mg/dl	=	Borderline High Blood Cholesterol
Over 240 mg/dl	=	High Blood Cholesterol

Studies show that people with high blood cholesterol are *four* times more likely to die of heart disease than people whose total cholesterol is under 200 mg/dl.

Interestingly, the number of people who have heart attacks whose total cholesterol is borderline is actually *greater* than the number in the high-risk group. Combined with other risk factors like smoking or high blood pressure, borderline high cholesterol can greatly increase chances of a heart attack. Many younger women are in this borderline group, and more of them than expected are developing heart disease. An estimated twenty-three thousand women under age sixty-five die of a heart attack each year; over one quarter of them are younger than fifty-five.

LDL Levels: According to the NCEP's new guidelines, an LDL reading above 160 mg/dl is now considered high-risk. Most people fall somewhere between 130 and 159 mg/dl, in the borderline category. The desirable level for LDL is less than 130 mg/dl.

People who have coronary heart disease (and are at risk of a recurrent episode) now have a lower LDL target level—100 mg/dl; the target had previously been 130 mg/dl.

HDL Versus LDL: The new guidelines also classify low HDL as a major risk factor for heart disease. Studies show that as many as 5 to 10 percent of Americans may be at increased risk for coronary artery disease solely because of *low* levels of HDL.

The danger zone for low HDL is considered to be below 45–35 mg/dl in women, since HDL appears to be more protective in women than men. Some 20 percent of heart attacks occur in people whose total cholesterol is below 200 mg/dl, but whose HDL is below 35. An HDL *above* 60 mg/dl is a "negative risk factor."

Triglycerides: The NCEP guidelines set the desirable level for TGL at under 200 mg/dl; borderline high TGL is 200–400 mg/dl, and high TGL ranges from 400 to 1,000 mg/dl.

However, recent studies have found triglycerides can also be a significant predictor of heart disease risk in women. Some experts now say the ideal level for TGL in a woman should be *under 100 mg/dl*. A twelve-year study of more than seven thousand men and women at ten medical centers around the country found coronary risk increased in women when TGL rose above 83 mg/dl, compared with 131 mg/dl for men, independent of other risk factors.

It should be noted that the "desirable" levels for total cholesterol, LDL and HDL were based on studies largely done in men. More research is needed to determine if the healthiest lipid levels for women are substantially different from those for men, especially for older women.

WHO NEEDS CHOLESTEROL TESTING?

In its revised guidelines, the National Cholesterol Education Program recommends that total cholesterol be measured at least once every five years in all adults of age twenty and over; HDL should be added to routine testing in a clinical setting.

According to James I. Cleeman, M.D., coordinator of the NCEP, this is a change from previous recommendations that HDL be tested only if total cholesterol is high. If tests show total cholesterol to be above 240 mg/dl, a complete "fasting" lipid breakdown (see page 63) measuring HDL, LDL and TGL is recommended. In addition, if HDL is below 35 mg/dl a lipid breakdown is also recommended.

"HDL and total cholesterol are used to predict the risk of coronary disease. If the risk is elevated, we use LDL as the index for whether a person might need to begin treatment. Then we need to know the levels of both HDL and LDL and, in some patients, the level of triglycerides, in order to tailor treatment. But lowering LDL is still the main goal of treatment," explains Dr. Cleeman.

People whose total cholesterol is borderline, but who have fewer than two coronary risk factors, would be given advice on diet and exercise and be tested again within a year. Those with borderline cholesterol, who have *two or more* cardiac risk factors, would be advised to have a complete lipid profile. People with previously diagnosed heart disease are at highest risk and need a fasting lipid breakdown as their initial test, says Dr. Cleeman. In addition, some experts recommend all adults with diabetes have

a lipid breakdown; diabetics may have higher amounts of fat in the blood.
The new guidelines also affect women in several areas:

• Age is now considered a risk factor. Age becomes a risk factor for women at age fifty-five; in men, the cutoff is age forty-five. So a woman over age fifty-five, who has borderline high cholesterol and *one* other cardiac risk factor would need a complete lipid breakdown.

• A premenopausal woman who has a high total cholesterol (even with no other cardiac risk factors) would need a complete lipid profile.

• The emphasis for treating high cholesterol in younger women would be on a cholesterol-lowering diet, weight loss and exercise; drug therapy would be delayed.

• After menopause (or in women with existing heart disease), a more aggressive treatment approach could be taken, including cholesterol-lowering drugs (see page 72).

Measuring Blood Fats: Total cholesterol and HDL can be measured at any time of the day, whether you have just eaten or not, but a complete lipid profile should only be done after fasting at least nine to twelve hours (with no alcohol for twenty-four hours). That's because LDL levels are actually estimated from a formula measuring other fats, including triglycerides, and food can cause a temporary rise in TGL. A new test has been approved to directly measure LDL.

Posture can also alter a cholesterol reading by affecting blood volume, so blood for a lipid breakdown is only drawn after a patient has been sitting down for at least five minutes. Total cholesterol can be measured by blood drawn from a finger-prick.

Be wary of walk-in cholesterol testing at places like shopping malls. The tests may not be as reliable as blood work performed in a laboratory, and they provide only a total cholesterol count, which will *not* evaluate your heart-disease risk as reliably as a test including HDL.

An over-the-counter home cholesterol testing kit was approved in 1993 by the U.S. Food and Drug Administration. Like shopping-mall tests, the kit measures only total cholesterol and may be of limited use for most people.

Women nearing the age of menopause should have their cholesterol checked when they have their regular physical. If there is a decline in

HDL or an increase in LDL, a special diet and exercise program can help remedy this, since exercise has been shown to raise HDL levels (see page 130). A 1993 study found women least likely to have their cholesterol tested are those who rely solely on a gynecologist for routine preventive care.

Should your LDL be between 130 and 159 mg/dl, doctors may advise watching your diet and starting an exercise program. Under the new guidelines, an LDL level above 160 will prompt a strict cholesterol-lowering diet.

RAYE'S STORY

"My sister has high cholesterol, my grandmother died of a stroke, and my father had a heart attack. When I hit menopause, I knew I should get my cholesterol tested. My cholesterol was nearly 300! That test changed my life.

"I'm not overweight. I'm sixty-three and semiretired. I used to be pretty active. But I wasn't getting a lot of exercise once I cut back on my working hours. Now I go walking every day.

"My husband loves steak and pot roast. But now I serve more chicken and fish and I always take the skin off the chicken. I also serve lots of fresh fruits and vegetables, skim milk and low-fat cheese.

"My husband has had to get used to that. At first, he complained incessantly. But now, he's come around. Especially since he's lost weight. And his cholesterol has come down, too. We're both under 200. I take credit for that!"

HOW CHANGING YOUR DIET
REDUCES YOUR RISK

Since eating saturated fat reduces the liver's ability to make more lipo-proteins to carry cholesterol to the bloodstream, reducing the amount of saturated fat in your diet will lower cholesterol.

There are two kinds of unsaturated fat: polyunsaturated fats and monounsaturated fats. Polyunsaturated fats contain linoleic acid, a key nutrient for cell formation and the functioning of the nervous system, which the body doesn't produce on its own. Monounsaturated fats are mostly oleic acid, and have been reported to lower blood pressure and blood glucose as well as blood cholesterol.

New studies suggest that LDL containing oleic acid may resist the oxidation that helps create "foam cells." High intakes of polyunsaturated fats generally lower both LDL and HDL, while monounsaturated fats lower LDL but leave HDL unchanged; olive oil may also raise HDL. A recent study found substituting olive oil for a polyunsaturated vegetable oil increased the ratio of HDL to LDL in women by 30 percent, compared with 17 percent in men. Another reason to eat more monounsaturated fats: Very high levels of linoleic acid in the diet have been linked to various types of cancers.

Polyunsaturated fats include vegetable oils like safflower, corn, soybean, cottonseed, sesame and sunflower. Olive oil, peanut and canola (or rapeseed) are high in monounsaturated fats.

Experts say overall fat intake should be *less* than 30 percent (perhaps as low as 25 to 20 percent) of a day's calories. No more than 7.5–10 percent of the day's fat calories should come from saturated fat; 10–15 percent should be monounsaturated fats and the remainder from polyunsaturated fat (see our fat-gram chart on page 256).

As you can see from the following chart of fats in cooking oils, when the amount of monounsaturated fat decreases, the amount of saturated fat soars.

FATS IN COOKING OILS

VEGETABLE OIL/ SHORTENING	SATURATED FAT %	POLYUNSATURATED FAT %	MONOUNSATURATED FAT %
Olive Oil	13	8	74
Canola Oil	7	33	55
Peanut Oil	17	32	46
Corn Oil	13	59	24
Soybean Oil	14	58	23
Sunflower Oil	10	66	20
Cottonseed Oil	26	52	18
Safflower Oil	9	75	12
Palm Kernel Oil	81	2	11
Coconut Oil	86	2	6

Source: The National Institutes of Health.

There are now low-fat (and nonfat) versions of many foods, as well as select cuts of beef available with as little saturated fat as skinless chicken. The key is reading food labels carefully, choosing those products lowest in fat and keeping track of how many grams of fat you eat each day. (More tips on cutting fat are in Chapter 6.)

While some experts have questioned the effectiveness of low-fat diets in women, a 1994 study from the Center for Human Nutrition at the University of Texas Southwestern Medical Center found benefits for women with high LDL cholesterol. The study of forty-one postmenopausal women found that those who followed a diet of 30 percent of calories from fat, 10 percent of calories from saturated fat and 300 mg of cholesterol per day lowered their LDL by an average of 11 mg/dl after three months (some reducing LDL by as much as 50 mg/dl). The study was small, and a few women had a small drop in HDL (3 mg/dl), with LDL reductions somewhat less than men would have achieved. But study director Margo A. Denke, M.D., believes that at least half of women with high cholesterol could lower LDL with a low-fat diet alone, avoiding the need for cholesterol-lowering drugs.

TRANS FATTY ACIDS

There is another type of dietary fat you need to be aware of: *trans fatty acids*. Trans fats are formed when liquid vegetable oils are *hydrogenated*— treated with hydrogen to make them solid (as in stick margarine or shortening) and to prevent spoilage. Hydrogenated vegetable oils are used to fry fast foods and are also found in commercial pies, cookies and cakes.

Recent studies show that trans fatty acids act just like saturated fat to raise artery-clogging LDL cholesterol while lowering HDL. One controversial report blames trans fats for thirty thousand deaths per year in this country.

An update from the Nurses' Health Study showed that women who ate four or more teaspoons a day of solid margarine may have a 50 percent greater risk of coronary disease than women who ate solid margarine only once a month. The risk rose to 70 percent if a woman ate six or more teaspoons of margarine a day. Surprisingly, the study found no increase in risk associated with butter (possibly because people eat it so sparingly these days).

News like this can be frustrating. First we were told that butter was bad; now we find out certain forms of margarine may be just as lethal! And by now you're wondering: "So what do I spread on my toast?" The answer: *ANY type of fat in excess is not good for you.* NYU cardiologist Dr. Stephen Siegel points out that consuming four to six teaspoons of margarine or vegetable oil a day is a lot of fat (and calories) to begin with. However, margarine is now the leading source of fat in American diets.

A 1994 advisory from the American Heart Association's Nutrition Committee says soft tub diet margarines (which contain more water and less trans fatty acids) are better for your heart than hard margarines. The AHA advisory recommends choosing margarine with no more than 2 grams of saturated fat per tablespoon, and limiting intake to five to eight teaspoons a day of *all* fats and oils. Or, try a tasty *no-fat* alternative: jelly.

When cooking, use oils in their original form, instead of shortening, and use less of them. Cooking sprays and nonstick pans are a good way to cut back on fat without sacrificing flavor.

CUTTING DOWN ON CHOLESTEROL

In addition to cutting fat, you need to watch the amount of cholesterol in your diet. Eating too many foods high in cholesterol will only add to what's already circulating in your blood. Cholesterol is found in animal products and should be limited to less than 300 milligrams a day.

Just one egg yolk contains about 270 milligrams of cholesterol, which is why eggs are always the first thing doctors tell you to cut back on if you need a low-cholesterol diet. Shellfish like shrimp and crabs also contain a lot of cholesterol, even though they're low in saturated fat. Three and a half ounces of cooked shrimp has about 195 milligrams of cholesterol.

But don't go crazy. You shouldn't feel that you *can't* have eggs (unless a doctor says so). You may have an egg, you may have cheese, you may have beef. Just eat them less often, in smaller quantities, and pick lower-fat versions. *Again, the key is moderation, not deprivation.*

If you need a cholesterol-lowering diet, you and your doctor might use the following diet guidelines from NYU teaching affiliate Lenox Hill Hospital to work out meal plans that are appropriate for you. The diet separates people into three risk categories—yellow, blue and green— based on their cholesterol levels and risk factors.

However, do not embark on any restrictive diet without consulting a physician first. For more information on the fat, cholesterol and other contents of foods, see Chapter 6.

SAMPLE CHOLESTEROL-MANAGEMENT DIETS

THE YELLOW DIET: For individuals with borderline high cholesterol (200–239 mg/dl) and no other cardiac risk factors. This diet is based on a maximum of 300 mg of cholesterol a day and no more than 30 percent of total calories from fat.

FOOD CHOICES	ALLOWED	AVOID
Milk Products	Skim milk, 99% low-fat milk, low-fat yogurt	Whole milk, condensed milk, chocolate milk, instant cocoa, nondairy creamers, cream (sour, heavy and whipped cream), whole-milk yogurt, eggnog, malted milk
Eggs	Egg yolks, limit one weekly; egg white	Whole eggs, egg yolks
Cheeses	Cheeses made from skim or part skim milk, low-fat cottage cheese, mozzarella, ricotta, farmer cheese; cheese with less than 5 grams fat per ounce	Cheeses made from whole milk or cream
Meat/Fish	Four ounces lean beef, pork, lamb and veal, three times a week; skinless chicken; shell-fish in moderation	Processed lunch meats, smoked cured meats (bacon, ham), frankfurters, sausage, corned beef, pastrami, spare-ribs, duck, organ meats, caviar, fish roe
Bread/Cereal	White, whole wheat rye and pumpernickel breads; bagels, English muffins, melba toast, pretzels, crackers, hot or dry cereal; air-popped, unbuttered popcorn	Commercial biscuits, muffins, doughnuts, sweet rolls, danish; butter rolls, corn chips, po-tato chips, commercial popcorn.
Starches	Potatoes, rice, pasta; noodles without cream or butter	Creamed or scalloped pota-toes; potatoes fried in satu-rated fat; rice mixes with cream sauces
Fruit	All fresh, frozen, canned, or dried fruit and fruit juices	

FOOD CHOICES	ALLOWED	AVOID
Vegetables	All fresh, frozen, or canned vegetables	Vegetables packed in butter or cream sauces
Fats (in limited amounts)	Margarine, peanut butter, nuts, mayonnaise, oils (corn, peanut, safflower, olive, canola); low-fat or fat-free salad dressings	Butter, lard, solid vegetable shortening, palm, coconut oils; commercial salad dressings, gravies, gravy made from meat; béarnaise and hollandaise sauce
Beverages	Coffee, tea, decaffeinated coffee and tea; alcohol (consult physician first)	
Desserts/Sugars	Sugar, jelly, jam, marmalade, pure sugar candy, gelatine, sherbet, fruit ice, angel food cake, vanilla wafers, ginger snaps, meringues; pies and puddings made with low-fat ingredients	Commercial cakes, pies, cookies, pastries, ice cream, ice milk, puddings, custards, chocolate, coconut, whipped cream desserts; candy made with butter, cream or coconut.
Soups	Homemade vegetable or meat stock; soups skimmed of fat; canned or instant soup without milk or cream; bouillon cubes	All creamed soups
Flavors/Spices	Herbs, spices, horseradish, Tabasco sauce, pickles, mustard, salt ketchup, barbecue sauce, soy sauce, Worcestershire sauce, relishes	Condiments or flavor aids made from fats and oils

THE BLUE DIET: for individuals with borderline high cholesterol plus two or more cardiac risk factors. This diet is based on a maximum of 150 milligrams of cholesterol a day, with no more than 25 percent of total calories from fat.

If your risk category is in the blue zone, use the yellow diet as a guide, but modify it as follows:

- Limit consumption of red meat to four to six ounces a week.
- Avoid all egg yolks and products made with egg yolks.
- Use cheese and milk with no more than 1 percent fat.

THE GREEN DIET: for individuals with high cholesterol, 240 mg/dl or higher. This diet is based on a maximum of 100 milligrams of cholesterol a day, with no more than 20 percent of calories from fat.

If your risk category is in the green zone, follow guidelines for the yellow and blue diets and, in addition:

- Eat only 3 ounces of poultry or fish per day.
- Consume mainly whole grains, legumes, vegetables and fruits.
- Avoid cheese.
- Use only skim milk.

FOR PATIENTS WITH HIGH TRIGLYCERIDES: In addition to limiting dietary fats, avoid simple sugars. These include:

- Table sugar
- Candy
- Cakes, pies, cookies
- Ice cream
- Sugared soda
- Fruit drinks, sugared gelatin

Source: *The Lenox Hill Hospital Guide to Managing Cholesterol.* Reprinted by permission.

ELLEN'S STORY

"I got my cholesterol tested about four years ago. I was feeling tired and washed out and I was having a lot of difficulty breathing. I was also overweight. I teach English at a small New England college, and when I'd be carrying books up the stairs, I'd get short of breath. There's nothing cute about having to have someone carry your books at my age.

"My cholesterol was 296. My doctor put me on a very low-fat diet immediately and told me to start exercising. He said if that didn't work, I'd need cholesterol-lowering drugs.

"The hardest thing for me was giving up ice cream. My parents had an old-fashioned ice-cream parlor, and I grew up eating as much of it as I wanted. I was sixty and still eating ice cream several times a week.

"Now I buy no-fat frozen yogurt and put fresh fruit on top. It's not the same as an ice cream sundae. But most of the time, I like it. Occasionally, I buy a small cone or cup of real ice cream for a treat, but not that often. I go walking several times a week with a friend. My weight has come down and my cholesterol is now close to 200. So the sacrifice was worth it."

WHAT ABOUT "CHOLESTEROL-
FIGHTING" FOODS?

Every few years, a new food or dietary supplement is touted as a "cholesterol fighter." Some of the recent candidates:

Garlic: A 1993 report in the Annals of Internal Medicine, reviewing five studies in the United States and Germany, suggested that eating the equivalent of one half to one clove of garlic a day could lower total blood cholesterol by about 9 percent in people with high serum cholesterol. The studies involved 365 people with serum cholesterol averaging 262–306 mg/dl. The participants ate garlic extract tablets or powders; the average reduction in cholesterol was 23 mg/dl.

This may be due to a chemical called polyphenols, found in garlic (and certain fruits and vegetables, as well as red wine). Polyphenols may help lower cholesterol and are believed to make blood platelets less sticky.

Psyllium: A study in the same issue of the Annals suggested the fiber supplement psyllium, taken twice daily, could produce a 6 percent drop in total cholesterol. The study, by Washington University School of Medicine in St. Louis, the University of Cincinnati, and Procter and Gamble (makers of Metamucil, a fiber supplement which happens to contain psyllium) say psyllium may also double chances of reducing LDL cholesterol.

Oat Bran: A 1992 overview in the Journal of the American Medical Association of a dozen studies on oat bran found that it does indeed fight cholesterol, but rather minimally. The analysis found that eating 3 grams a day of ready-to-eat oat bran cereal (about three packets of instant oatmeal) reduced total blood cholesterol between 5 and 6 milligrams per deciliter. That amounts to a 2 to 3 percent decline for people with borderline cholesterol.

Soluble fibers like oat bran or psyllium form a gel in the intestine, trapping cholesterol and preventing it from being reabsorbed by the body (see page 120). Scientists have also found that taking fiber supplements enlarges LDL particles; smaller, denser LDL particles are more harmful (women seem protected from this harmful LDL until after menopause).

Other possible cholesterol-fighting foods may be carrots and dried beans. Researchers at the U.S. Department of Agriculture say calcium pectate, contained in the cell walls of carrots, may speed up the way our body gets rid of cholesterol. Dried beans are thought to slow production of cholesterol in the body.

*But experts stress that there is no food or food supplement that will provide
a quick fix to lower high cholesterol.* By making long-term dietary changes,
eating less fat and more fiber, some individuals could lower their blood
cholesterol by as much as 10 to 20 percent. For every 1 percent drop in
cholesterol, your risk of a heart attack also drops by 2 to 3 percent!

HOW EXERCISE AND
WEIGHT LOSS HELP

The new cholesterol-treatment guidelines emphasize physical activity and
weight loss, since they enhance diet therapy. When we exercise, the body
takes its energy first from circulating glucose and triglycerides. As we
exercise, triglycerides go down, HDL goes up—*and* we lose weight!

Five to ten pounds of weight loss can actually *double* the LDL reduction achieved by cutting back on saturated fat and cholesterol. In fact, a
1994 study from the Baylor College of Medicine finds that losing 5 pounds
on a low-fat diet can translate into as much as a 10 percent reduction in
total cholesterol! Losing weight also reduces other coronary risk factors
like blood pressure and glucose intolerance.

In addition, a recent study from the University of Pittsburgh shows
that regular exercise slows the decline in HDL and prevents formation of
an HDL component called *HDL 2* that occurs in women after menopause.
These changes appeared to be independent of body weight, and a woman's
HDL decline was slowed even if she *didn't* lose weight. For more on the
benefits of exercise and a sample walking program, see Chapter 7.

CHOLESTEROL-LOWERING DRUGS

Recent studies show that, for some people with high LDL, diet and exercise may *not* appreciably lower their cholesterol.

If a really strict low-fat diet (no more than 200 milligrams of cholesterol and a scant 7 percent of calories from fat) and an exercise program
fail to lower cholesterol in six to twelve months, doctors may consider
using cholesterol-lowering drugs.

According to the National Cholesterol Education Program's updated
treatment guidelines, candidates and goals for drug therapy include:

• Adults whose LDL remains at 190 mg/dl or higher, with fewer than two risk factors. Target LDL: 160 mg/dl.

• Individuals whose LDL is 160 mg/dl, with two or more risk factors. Target LDL: 130 mg/dl.

• People with established coronary disease whose LDL is above 130 mg/dl. Target LDL: 100 mg/dl or lower.

• Premenopausal women with unusually high LDL or multiple coronary risk factors might be considered for drug therapy.

"However, for premenopausal women with LDL between 190 and 220 and no other risk factors, the use of drugs would generally be delayed, except in high-risk patients such as those with diabetes," explains the NCEP's Dr. Cleeman. "Under the new guidelines, estrogen replacement may be prescribed instead of cholesterol-lowering drugs in some women."

A combination of diet, drugs and exercise can result in an average reduction in cholesterol levels of 20 percent, lowering a woman's chance of a heart attack considerably. In some patients, combining two cholesterol-lowering drugs may reduce LDL alone by 40 to 50 percent. Preliminary studies also suggest aggressive cholesterol-lowering therapy can make diseased coronary arteries behave more like healthy ones!

The information below details the major types of cholesterol-lowering drugs and how they work.

CHOLESTEROL-LOWERING DRUGS

STATINS/HMG CoA REDUCTASE INHIBITORS: These drugs, including lovastatin (Mevacor) and fluvastatin sodium (Lescol) increase the body's ability to remove cholesterol from the blood. They do this by blocking *HMG CoA reductase,* an enzyme essential for cholesterol formation, so that the body makes less cholesterol and takes more of what it needs from the blood. Statins are very effective and can reduce LDL by as much as 40 percent. In higher doses, they may also slightly reduce triglycerides and boost HDL. One study suggests statins may actually *shrink* atherosclerotic plaques.

Potential Side Effects: Side effects include dizziness, headaches, muscle pain and some stomach discomfort. The drug may also cause liver dysfunction, so periodic liver function tests are needed.

Resin Drugs: Also called "bile acid sequestrants," this class of drugs includes cholestyramine (Questran) and colestipol (Colestid). Resin drugs trap bile-containing cholesterol in the digestive tract and then carry it out of the body. This helps cholesterol levels, because the body would normally reabsorb the bile (and the cholesterol in it). Since the liver needs cholesterol to produce bile, it will remove new cholesterol (especially LDL) from the blood for this purpose.

Resin drugs would only be prescribed for someone with high LDL and normal triglycerides, because they may raise TGL in some people.

Potential Side Effects: Since resin drugs may be taken with meals, side effects can include upset stomach, vomiting, occasional constipation or heartburn. They may also interfere with absorption of other heart medications, including thiazide diuretics, warfarin, digoxin and beta blockers.

Fibric-Acid Derivatives: Fibric acids like gemfibrozil (Lopid) enhance metabolism of cholesterol, reduce levels of triglycerides and raise HDL. They work by breaking down VLDLs in the blood.

Potential Side Effects: Side effects include diarrhea, nausea, flatulence and sometimes vomiting.

Nicotinic Acid: Nicotinic acid, or niacin, is a B vitamin and is believed to slow formation of cholesterol from fatty acids in the liver by lowering production of VLDL. Niacin (lipo-nicin, nicobid) also lowers triglyceride levels and is one of the few drugs that can also increase HDL.

Potential Side Effects: Side effects from nicotinic acid include severe redness of face and body, itching and gastrointestinal distress. It can also cause liver abnormalities and abnormal heart rhythms. Niacin is usually started in low doses and increased slowly over several weeks to minimize these side effects, since larger amounts are needed to be effective.

Warning: Niacin is not a prescription drug and is available in health food stores. Taken in the doses needed to lower cholesterol, niacin drugs can have serious side effects and should *never* be taken without a physician's approval.

Probucol (Lorelco): Probucol is a member of a fairly new class of cholesterol-lowering drugs that work by changing the makeup of LDL. It inhibits the oxidation of LDL particles, preventing them from forming plaques and allowing LDL to be removed more quickly from the bloodstream. New studies say the drug is effective, even when cholesterol levels are high. However, Probucol also *lowers* HDL.

Potential Side Effects: Minor side effects may include indigestion and occasional diarrhea, as well as rashes and insomnia.

Sources: *Physicians' Desk Reference, 1993*; National Cholesterol Education Program, *Second Report of Adult Treatment, Panel II, 1993.*

CHOLESTEROL-LOWERING DRUGS
AND WOMEN

The *first* major study of women and cholesterol drug therapy, reported back in 1991, concluded that these drugs work just as well for women as they do for men. Almost thirty-four hundred women participated in the EXCEL study of the statin drug lovastatin conducted at 362 medical centers across the country. All of the women were put on low-fat, low-cholesterol diets and were randomly assigned to various doses of lovastatin or to a placebo. The study found lovastatin lowered LDL cholesterol in 40 to 87 percent of women considered high risk (those with existing heart disease or two or more risk factors). The greatest reduction was in women over age sixty-five, whose risk of heart disease is highest.

In 1994, Researchers in the Canadian Coronary Atherosclerosis Intervention Trial reported that lovastatin can also *slow* the progression of coronary disease and even *prevent* the development of new plaques. The two-year randomized trial of 331 men and women diagnosed with atherosclerosis found that even small doses of the drug were equally successful in men and women in slowing further narrowing of the coronary arteries.

Other studies show that atherosclerosis in women can even be *reversed* with drug and diet therapy. Researchers at the University of California at San Francisco followed forty-one women and thirty-one men treated over two years for a form of familial hypercholesterolemia. The study found diet therapy along with a combination of three drugs (colestipol, niacin and lovastatin) produced bigger reductions in LDL cholesterol and arterial plaques than diet alone and smaller doses of one or two drugs. The lower the LDL went, the greater the improvement. In fact, the intensively treated women had *better* results than the men.

CAN ATHEROSCLEROSIS BE REVERSED?

There is some evidence that drastic diet and lifestyle changes can actually reverse atherosclerosis. A "reversal" program developed by Dean Ornish, M.D., director of the Preventive Medicine Research Institute in Sausalito, California, calls for a vegetarian diet with no more than 10 percent of calories from fat; daily exercise; stress management through yoga and meditation; and participation in a support group to help patients stick to these lifestyle changes.

After a year on the program, patients with severe coronary disease reduced arterial plaques by about 10 percent and lowered their cholesterol by 40 percent; after four years, the patients reduced plaques even further, resulting in improved blood flow to the heart. Similar programs are being established around the country. However, this is a very strict regimen and experts say otherwise healthy people who simply have elevated cholesterol would find it hard to stick with it.

CHOLESTEROL-LOWERING SURGERY

If medication and a strict low-fat diet fail to reduce excessively high cholesterol, surgery may be performed as a last resort. The surgery, called an *ileal bypass*, involves making an incision in the abdomen and bypassing the bottom portion of the small intestine, where cholesterol from food and from bile secreted by the liver is absorbed. The cholesterol is not absorbed into the blood, but is excreted from the body instead.

For men and women whose cholesterol levels put them at extremely high risk of a heart attack, an ileal bypass may result in a 40 percent reduction in cholesterol and 60 percent fewer coronary bypass operations.

The good news is that, for most women, high cholesterol can be controlled with a combination of dietary changes, weight loss and regular exercise. And a woman at especially high risk of a heart attack will benefit from aggressive cholesterol-lowering therapy.

5

Pare Down Your Body Fat

WHEN YOU STEPPED on the scale this morning, did you wince at what you saw? You're not alone. A recent report found that one third of American women weigh more than they should.

If you have no other cardiac risk factors, those few extra pounds will *not* affect your health. It's having a large amount of *excess* weight that gets you into trouble. Women who do not need to lose weight may find this chapter helpful in making eating habits healthier.

Women who are obese—20 percent or more over the normal weight for their height and build—have a *doubled* risk for heart disease and hypertension at any given age, even if they have no other risk factors for coronary heart disease.

But dieting is not the answer; overly restricting what you eat is actually a barrier to weight control. You need to make permanent changes in the way you eat that will lead to a healthy weight—and *that* will make a big difference to your heart.

DO YOU NEED TO LOSE WEIGHT?

In 1990, the U.S. Department of Health and Human Services and the U.S. Department of Agriculture issued new guidelines for a "healthy

weight." This new concept is designed to replace the culturally determined notion of "ideal" or "desirable" body weight (which is often
unrealistically low), by looking at a person's health as well as actual
pounds of body weight.* The new table of acceptable weights makes
no distinction by sex; women should generally be in the lower weight
ranges.**

There are three factors to consider in determining if you need to
lose weight:

• Do you have any health problems related to weight which could
be improved by weight loss?

• Is most of your weight distributed around your abdomen (an
"apple" body shape)?

• Do you weigh more than the acceptable range for your height
and age?

Check the following statements that apply to you, and add up the
number of "yes" answers to get your health score. Then measure your
waist-to-hip ratio and consult the weight table below. If your score is
low, your waist-to-hip ratio acceptable, and you're within normal
weight ranges, you don't need to lose weight for medical reasons.

PART ONE

1. Do you have "high normal" or high blood pressure? Yes _____
   No _____

2. Is your cholesterol above 200 mg/dl? Yes _____ No

3. Do you have diabetes? Yes _____ No _____

4. Do you have a family history of diabetes? Yes _____ No _____

*Note: If you wish to lose weight for cosmetic reasons, experts at
NYU suggest the best way to pick a goal is to look back on what
you've weighed over the years and find the weight that was easiest
for you to maintain, rather than your lowest weight.

**This does not imply that it's good or desirable to gain weight
after age 35. Recent studies suggest that even modest weight gains
in midlife can increase heart risk. Women over 35 should be at the
lower end or even slightly below the suggested weights.

5. Do you have a family history of heart disease? Yes _____
   No _____

6. Do you have a sedentary lifestyle? Yes _____ No _____

7. Do you frequently eat junk food, full-fat dairy products, fried foods,
   fatty red meats? Yes _____ No _____

8. Do you gain weight in times of stress, then frantically try to lose it
   again? Yes _____ No _____

PART TWO

To figure out your waist-to-hip ratio, use a tape measure to measure
your waist and hips. Now divide your waist measurement by your hip
measurement. If you end up with 0.75 or greater, you're "apple"
shaped. If the result is less than 0.75, you're "pear" shaped.

For example, a 32-inch waist divided by 38-inch hips would be
0.84, apple-shaped. A 29-inch waist divided by 40-inch hips is 0.72,
definitely pear-shaped.

The higher your waist-to-hip ratio, the higher your risk for heart
disease and other health problems.

Waist measurement _____ divided by hip measurement _____
equals _____. _____, your waist-to-hip ratio.

PART THREE
ACCEPTABLE WEIGHTS FOR MEN AND WOMEN

HEIGHT	WEIGHT (LBS)	HEIGHT	WEIGHT
	19–34 Years		34 years and up
5'0"	97–128	5'0"	108–138
5'1"	101–132	5'1"	111–143
5'2"	104–137	5'2"	115–148
5'3"	101–141	5'3"	119–152
5'4"	111–146	5'4"	122–157
5'5"	114–150	5'5"	126–162
5'6"	118–155	5'6"	130–167
5'7"	121–160	5'7"	134–172
5'8"	125–164	5'8"	138–178
5'9"	129–169	5'9"	142–183

HEIGHT	WEIGHT (LBS)	HEIGHT	WEIGHT
	19–34 Years		34 years and up
5'10"	132–174	5'10"	146–188
5'11"	136–179	5'11"	151–194
6'0"	140–184	6'0"	155–199

Your height: _____Your weight: _____
Your waist-to-hip ratio: _____ : _____
Your health score: _____

Source: USDA/DHHS *Dietary Guidelines for Americans,* Third Edition, 1990.

WHY FAT CAN BE A KILLER

The Nurses' Health Study has found that 70 percent of coronary heart disease in obese women (and 40 percent of heart disease in all women) can be directly attributed to excess body fat. This is true for women of all ages, but especially for women *under age fifty.* If an overweight woman also smokes, she's five times more likely to have heart disease as a woman of the same weight who doesn't smoke.

Actually, experts now say the problem is not really just pounds, but the percentage of excess body fat and where the fat is distributed. The belly fat that gives you an "apple" shape, and the fat on the hips and thighs that makes you "pear" shaped—act differently in the body.

New research has confirmed that being an "apple" can increase your risk of heart disease and certain cancers. Fat cells on the buttocks and thighs are called *hyperplastic.* They are found directly under the skin, are small and numerous and are used more for storage of energy, such as when you're pregnant or breast-feeding. But when a woman isn't pregnant, this type of fat isn't as metabolically active, so it doesn't break down as easily, and is harder to get rid of.

Fat cells found in the upper body and abdomen are called *hypertrophic.* They're larger, fewer in number, and they shrink more when you lose weight. Abdominal fat is more involved in day-to-day regulation of energy, breaking down in response to different signals from our hormones and nervous system.

When this fat breaks down, it generates "free fatty acids" that travel to the liver and stimulate production of triglycerides, which in turn lower levels of HDL, the good cholesterol, explains John Crouse, M.D., a professor of medicine at the Bowman Gray School of Medicine in Winston-Salem, North Carolina.

Dr. Crouse has found that apple-shaped women generate even more dangerous triglycerides after eating. These extra fatty acids from belly fat also reduce the breakdown of insulin by the liver, adds Dr. Crouse. This increases levels of insulin in the blood, possibly leading to insulin resistance and also increasing the risk of diabetes.

Fat cells may increase a woman's estrogen levels, which can affect the way the body uses insulin. So you can see why being overweight and having diabetes are *bigger* risk factors for heart disease in women than in men. And even though an overweight "apple" and "pear" may weigh the same, the extra upper body fat makes the "apple"-shaped woman more likely to die at an earlier age from cardiovascular disease.

Smokers also tend to have more upper body fat than nonsmokers, possibly because of the influence of chemicals in cigarette smoke on hormones.

The good news is that if you have a favorable waist-to-hip ratio, experts say you may not even have to lose those few extra pounds around your hips. If you have *no* other risk factors for cardiovascular disease and if you exercise regularly, you will still be healthier, even though you may technically weigh a bit more than you should.

In addition, when you lose weight, you generally lose it fastest from the tummy, helping to get rid of the "apple" shape and lower your risk for both heart disease and cancer.

CAN YOU BLAME IT ON GENES?

Women are programmed to gain weight in the hips and thighs, while men tend to put on pounds around their middles. When women lose estrogen at menopause, the small amounts of male hormones in their bodies may trigger weight gain around their middle.

You can also blame your family tree for those "love handles." Studies show that 80 percent of children with two overweight parents become fat.

Recently, scientists at the University of California at Los Angeles isolated a gene that triggers production of a protein called *lipoprotein lipase,* which helps the body store fat. The researchers at the Cedars Sinai Medical Center in Los Angeles say this may explain why overweight people find it hard to keep off weight once they've lost it. When obese people lose weight, their lipoprotein lipase levels rise and the levels stay high, even after the weight is lost, making it hard to keep pounds from creeping back.

Children of overweight parents may also be born with a higher than normal number of fat cells or larger fat cells, which increases the amount of fat the body can store. And some people simply store extra calories as fat, whereas others burn it up more easily. This may help to explain why people reach weight plateaus. Your body may be programmed to weigh a certain amount and will resist your attempts to go below that level. Repeated dieting can slow metabolism and make weight loss even harder. So for some people, maintaining a healthy weight level, rather than weight loss, may be the key to heart health.

CELIA'S STORY

"You know what I want? I'm a size 22 and I want to be a size 18 again. Now that may seem large to you, but that's the size I want to be. I was able to maintain that size. I always felt good when I was that size: big and healthy. I was a size 16 once; size 16 is not me. I don't want to be skinny, don't want to be no scrawny-looking sister with chicken-wing arms."

RACIAL AND SOCIAL FACTORS

According to the Coronary Artery Risk Development in Young Adults (CARDIA) study, 30 percent of African-American women ages eighteen to thirty are obese, compared to 14 percent of white women. About half of Native-American and Mexican-American women are obese. By ages forty-five to sixty-five, 77 percent of black women can be considered obese, compared to about half of white women. A 1994 update from the CARDIA study also found that all women gain weight after a first pregnancy and many continue to gain, but black women put on more pounds than their white counterparts.

For black women, obesity can show up early in life. The National Heart, Lung and Blood Institute's Growth and Health Study, which is following the development of 2,379 healthy girls in three urban areas, found that African-American girls have greater amounts of body fat and higher blood pressure as early as age nine, which puts them at two to four times greater risk of developing heart disease as adults, compared with white girls their age.

An increased prevalence of obesity is believed to be partly responsible for the higher incidence of diabetes and hypertension among blacks, as well as among Native-American women.

Why are so many women of color overweight? A woman's level of income, her social situation, food preferences and differing cultural attitudes about eating and body image all play a role.

A 1991 report in the journal *Women & Health*, which reviewed available studies on obesity, gender, poverty and race, concluded that women of color, particularly poor black and Latina women, are six times more likely to be overweight than middle-class white women. The report cited a number of contributing factors directly relating to poverty: lack of control over life choices and opportunities; a sense of fatalism; the stress of poverty and of racism; low-paying jobs; a need for instant gratification; and less concern about overeating.

Struggling with the time pressures and responsibilities of working, home and children, many women turn to convenience foods as a quick way to feed their families. Most convenience foods are high in fat, and fat-laden fast foods are aggressively marketed in poor or minority communities. Many women may be unaware that they can prepare lower-fat versions of favorite ethnic dishes.

In addition, diet programs and health clubs are more accessible to higher-income women, and fear of crime may scare women away from outdoor exercise in poorer neighborhoods.

Moreover, eating practices and foods have different meanings within different cultural groups. The idea of expressing abundance, love and community through food are all bound up in our eating habits. In many ethnic groups and cultures, setting a good table remains a measure of womanliness.

Certain dishes high in fat and calories are staples among different ethnic groups: deep-fried foods like fried chicken; butter "smothered" okra, pasta or enchiladas stuffed with cheese; beans refried in lard, fat-based gravies, butter-laden pastries and cakes. Under certain circumstances, refusing such foods might be construed as rejecting those who offer them. Is there *any* woman who hasn't eaten more than she intended at a holiday gathering because she didn't want to hurt someone's feelings?

These same foods become "comfort foods" in times of stress or emotional upset. We also "reward" ourselves with those foods. Those are *universal* reasons why women overeat, which cut across social, racial and cultural lines.

Various ethnic and racial groups also have different perceptions of what is "overweight." For most middle- and upper-class white women, being slender is equated with being healthy. But in many cultures and ethnic groups, being well-fleshed is considered a sign of good health. For example, Mexican Americans traditionally believe that being big, or *robusto*, makes a person more resistant to disease.

Linda Curtis O'Bannon, M.D., editor and publisher of *Urban Physician's Focus*, a minority healthcare newsletter, and a staff physician at the Humana-Michael Reese Hospital in Chicago, points out that historically, obesity symbolized wealth, social prestige, fertility and good health in societies where food wasn't always plentiful. "In Nigeria, adolescent daughters of the wealthy were sent into seclusion in special 'fattening huts' to make them more pleasing to prospective husbands," she notes.

Many overweight women say they are perfectly happy with the way they look and don't see obesity as a sign of ill health. But pile too many excess pounds on top of other risk factors and it adds up to a health threat.

While it's not possible to change one's genes, ethnicity or often one's social situation, it is possible to do something about this particular risk factor for heart disease.

We're not talking about becoming fashion-magazine thin or trying to alter your body to suit someone else's idea of beautiful; a woman can be a perfectly healthy size 16.

But if you also have a family history of high blood pressure, diabetes or other coronary risk factors, *losing as little as ten to fifteen pounds* can make a big difference to your heart. If you're overweight, just a 5 percent weight loss reduces your chances of developing high blood pressure by 50 percent. That's a big gain for so little!

WINNING AT LOSING

First, banish the word *diet* from your vocabulary. It is possible to achieve a 5 to 10 percent reduction in body weight over a year (a level that's not hard to maintain) using a sensible approach to weight loss.

To lose one pound of body fat, you need a deficit of 3,500 calories. For a sensible weight loss of a pound a week, that means most people simply need to eat 500 calories fewer per day, burn off 500 calories a day in exercise, or some combination of the two. (For *smaller* women, 500 calories may be a big chunk of a day's calories, so they may need to cut back by only 300 calories.)

There are basically seven keys to losing weight that are effective for most women, says NYU senior nutritionist Jennifer Stack.

First: Since fat is the most concentrated source of calories, cut back on fat. The body converts 90 percent of the fat we eat into body fat. But it has to work harder to convert complex carbohydrates like bread or pasta, so only 25 percent of those calories end up as stored body fat. Reduce fat intake to less than a third of your day's calories and replace it with complex carbohydrates and fiber like rice, pasta or beans if you're trying to lose.

Second: Keep close track of what you eat. Most overweight people eat more than they think they do. Researchers at the Weight Control Unit at St. Lukes-Roosevelt Hospital Center in New York questioned obese people who had failed at many diets about how much they ate each day. Most claimed they ate only about 1,100 calories a day. But when they were asked to keep food diaries, the records showed their actual calorie intake was at least twice that amount!

Third: Start a program of regular aerobic exercise (see Chapter 7). Aerobic exercise—any rhythmic, sustained activity that uses large groups of muscles—forces the body to mobilize stored fat as energy and raises the metabolism for hours afterward. Even a brisk walk around your block in a pair of comfortable old sweats will help you become more fit. But always consult a doctor before starting an exercise program.

Fourth: Lose weight gradually. Since an overweight person may have an enzymatic trigger for regaining lost weight, shedding pounds very slowly over a longer period of time may not set off this trigger or may produce a less extreme reaction.

Fifth: Don't ask your body to do more than it's capable of doing. Because of a woman's body composition (more fat tissue than a man's) and her metabolism (slower than a man's), most women will only lose between a half pound and a pound and a half a week.

Sixth: Start seeing yourself as a more fit individual, as an attractive, energetic woman who has control over what she eats and how she looks.

Seventh: Do not crash diet.

JOYCE'S STORY

"When I look in the mirror, I've never been happy with what I see. My weight has gone up and down all my life; mostly up. I gained a lot of weight with each child—and I've had four.

"I'm really big, a size 24, so when I read about this liquid diet program, I thought, 'That's for me.' And I lost weight like gangbusters. In the first month and a half, I lost eighteen pounds. So I thought, 'Great, I don't need to diet anymore.' I gained back that eighteen pounds and another four on top of it. I just couldn't stop eating.

"My husband says he likes me the way I am, but my doctor says it's unhealthy. I have high blood pressure and borderline diabetes. I have to watch what I eat now, and my doctor wants me to lose weight. But I really don't know how. I feel kind of desperate. I've been dieting all my life, and I'm sick of it. There has got to be another way."

CRASH DIETING
AND YOUR HEART

Semistarvation diets or unsupervised very low-calorie liquid diets may cause heart damage. Very low-calorie intake can result in dehydration, dangerous mineral imbalances and a drop in blood pressure from lack of adequate fluids. Essential minerals like potassium, called electrolytes, help regulate the electrical system in the heart, keeping its rhythm steady. Long-term complications of electrolyte imbalances include the risk of severe ventricular arrhythmias, which can be fatal.

In addition, people who are not terribly overweight who go on extreme diets for long periods start to lose lean body mass (muscle) along with the fat. This includes muscle tissue in the heart, which can damage the heart as well as other organs.

Data from the Framingham Heart Study found that people who take off weight, then put it back on, then frantically try to take it off again year after year are twice as likely to die of coronary heart disease. Thus, yo-yo dieting may be just as dangerous as remaining obese.

Experts speculate that when a person gains back a lot of fat (especially abdominal fat) after a diet, it may flood the liver with fatty acids, accelerating the process of atherosclerosis. In addition, factors that influence heart disease such as blood cholesterol levels, blood pressure and blood sugar will fluctuate with weight gained and lost and you may end up worse than you were to start out with.

EATING DISORDERS AND HEART DAMAGE

Surveys show that half of all American women diet at one time or another during a given year, and many don't even need to. Many of these constant dieters have a problem with body image, not fatty tissue.

A distorted sense of body image may lead to anorexia, an eating disorder in which a woman starves herself, or bulimia, where a woman gorges on food, then forces herself to vomit, abuses diuretics or laxatives or uses excessive exercise to purge herself of the excess calories. More than 90 percent of those afflicted with these eating disorders are adolescent and young-adult women.

Eating disorders can be deadly: One in ten cases of eating disorders leads to death from starvation, cardiac arrest or suicide. In women with anorexia (especially the binge-purge type) dehydration lowers blood volume, and starvation leads to loss of essential minerals called *electrolytes*, which help regulate the heart's electrical system, causing severe cardiac arrhythmias. When body fat has been depleted, anorexics begin to lose lean body mass, including vital muscle tissue in the heart. Women who suffer from anorexia and bulimia need prompt medical and psychiatric help.

TREATING OBESITY

More and more experts view some cases of obesity as a disease that may benefit from medical attention and treatment.

A four-year randomized trial from the University of Rochester School of Medicine found that appetite suppressants containing the drugs *fenfluramine* and *phentermine* can help morbidly obese people lose weight and keep it off as long as they take the drugs.

Fenfluramine (Pondimin) is a drug that boosts the amount of a brain chemical called *serotonin*, which suppresses appetite and makes people eat more slowly. Phentermine (Fastin) has effects similar to amphetamines— it makes people eat less but eat more rapidly. In the study, low doses of both drugs were given together.

Experts say these drugs are definitely *not* for people who want to shed ten pounds. These drugs do have side effects, such as dry mouth, dizziness, jitteriness and diarrhea. The U.S. Food and Drug Administration has approved these drugs for short-term use, but there's no information on their long-term safety.

DO YOU NEED A WEIGHT-LOSS PROGRAM?

For some women, losing weight is easier in a group setting. Consider joining a weight-loss program in your neighborhood, so transportation won't be a problem.

Nationally available weight-loss programs combine group meetings, limited nutritional education and "maintenance" sessions to help people try to avoid regaining weight. These programs also offer (sometimes require you to purchase) special prepackaged foods, which can increase their cost substantially.

Unfortunately, even with group support, most people tend to put the pounds back on unless they stay in the program a long time and *permanently change their eating habits and lifestyle.*

Before you sign up for any supervised weight-loss program, you need a complete physical and an electrocardiogram to make sure your heart is healthy. If your doctor finds a problem, you may need more specific dietary guidance than these programs can provide.

If you just need to lose between ten and fifteen pounds, avoid any weight-loss plan that restricts caloric intake to fewer than 1,000 calories a day. This reduces the chances of lowering your metabolism while you diet (regular exercise helps, too).

Also, forget those "liquid diets." A study by the Obesity Research Group at the University of Pennsylvania compared metabolism changes of women who went on a very low-calorie liquid diet of 420 calories a day to those of women who went on a diet of conventional food totaling 1,200 calories a day. During the first five weeks of the diet, the liquid dieters' metabolism dropped 21 percent, while the metabolisms of women on a conventional food diet fell only 10 percent. The liquid dieters' metabolism rebounded after they started eating regular food, resulting in weight gain.

In general, experts recommend medically supervised liquid diets (using protein and egg-based powders) of 400 to 800 calories a day *only* for people who are morbidly obese (that is, 100 percent or 100 pounds over their ideal body weight), who have been examined by a physician and who have a healthy electrocardiogram.

A liquid diet amounts to a modified fast, so there should be qualified medical supervision to make sure there's no dangerous loss of electrolytes during the diet, which can lead to heartbeat disturbances. Obesity experts warn people *never* to try this kind of liquid diet on their own; these programs are considered safe for heart patients, but *only* with medical supervision.

A WEIGHT-MANAGEMENT PROGRAM FOR WOMEN

Instead of a temporary diet, experts agree you need to adopt habits that restructure your eating habits for good. The Weight Management Program for Women at NYU Medical Center is designed to do just that.

"Moderation not deprivation" is the motto of the program, and it's probably the best advice for anyone trying to shed excess pounds or to break unhealthful eating habits.

The program is *not* a "diet" with forbidden foods and strict food regimens. Rather, it's an education in healthful eating. In the course, NYU senior nutritionist Jennifer Stack stresses that there are no "bad" foods, even fat (in fact, you need a small amount of fat in your diet to remain healthy). When you label a food you like as being "bad" for you and try to eliminate it from your diet, it just makes you feel deprived.

The emphasis is on learning what foods are "worth" nutritionally, and how to plan meals that will help you lose weight without feeling deprived. Participants set *achievable* weight goals, learn to recognize triggers for over-eating, and are also encouraged to begin a program of regular exercise. They also learn stress-management techniques (see Chapter 8) and behavior modification.

The first step is to select a *realistic* weight goal and a corresponding amount of daily calories needed to reach and maintain a healthy weight. The formula is simple: Multiply your weight goal by ten, and round off to the nearest hundred. The resulting number is the minimum number of calories you need to attain that goal.

Let's say you want to weigh 135 pounds:

$$\begin{array}{r} 135 \text{ pounds weight goal} \\ \underline{\times 10} \\ 1,350 = 1,400 \text{ calories per day} \end{array}$$

The next step is to provide a simple framework to create livable eating plans.

USING THE FOOD "EXCHANGE" CONCEPT

For meal planning, NYU's program uses the food "exchanges" established by the American Dietetic Association and the American Diabetes Association. Although the exchanges were designed primarily for diabetics, the system is based on principles of good nutrition that *anyone* can use.

There are six basic exchange groups: starches/breads, meats/proteins (including cheese), vegetables, fruits, milk and fats. Foods within each category are alike nutritionally—they contain approximately the same amount of carbohydrates, protein, fat and calories per portion. Each portion should be weighed or measured initially, to help you learn portion control.

For example, a slice of bread weighing one ounce counts as one bread exchange. One bread exchange contains approximately fifteen grams of carbohydrate, three grams of protein, a trace of fat and 80 calories. So if

you're making a sandwich for lunch, you might use up two bread exchanges, two or three meat exchanges and a fat exchange.

The emphasis is on a diet low in fat and rich in starches, fruits and
vegetables. Participants are encouraged to choose from lower-fat meats,
poultry and fish and to limit high-fat choices to fewer than three helpings
per week.

The following are lists of food exchanges per day for each calorie level,
based on the calorie and food exchange formula used in NYU's Weight
Management Program for Women. It's similar to the U.S. Department of
Agriculture's "Food Pyramid" plan for a healthful diet, but the number
of servings depends on the calories needed to lose weight.

NYU DAILY FOOD-EXCHANGE/CALORIE PLAN

FOOD GROUP	CALORIE LEVELS								
	1,100	1,200	1,300	1,400	1,500	1,600	1,700	1,800	1,900
Milk (1% fat or skim)	1½	2	2	2	2	2	2	2	2
Vegetables	3	3	3	3	3	3	3	3	3
Fruit	2	2	3	4	4	4	5	5	5
Bread/starch	5	5	5	5	6	6	6	7	8
Meat/protein	5	5	5	5	5	6	7	7	7
Fat	½	1½	2½	3½	4	4	4	4	4

Source: NYU Medical Center Health Education Center.

Over time, participants are encouraged to break free from rigidity of
the exchange in small steps. For example, you might create your own
version of a meal each day, then two meals. This helps you develop an
eating plan that's enjoyable and doable in the long run. Charts detailing
each food exchange group and listing the general types of foods and portions in each category are found in Appendix I. These are the same
exchange lists given to cardiac rehabilitation patients at NYU Medical
Center who need to lose weight.

Stack encourages people to build their first week's menus around the
sample menus outlined below, measuring and weighing portions. This
way, you'll get to see what three ounces of fish actually looks like and
whether you want to eat more of your starch exchanges for dinner, rather

than for lunch. People who loathe cereal can substitute half a bagel for breakfast; those who hate orange juice might have fruit instead, and so forth. After the first week or so on this regimen, the exchanges and sample menus become a general guideline for weight-loss meal planning and healthful eating.

Stack points out that while most of these meals are filling, some people may not feel satisfied. For example, some people feel that dinner is not quite complete without some sort of sweet. Don't deprive yourself of that sweet. Simply save up the exchange from another meal. No food is actually "forbidden," even pizza. (Cheese pizza is considered a "combination" food. One quarter of a ten-inch pizza combines two starch servings, one meat and one fat exchange. So one slice of cheese pizza along with fruit can be a perfectly acceptable lunch.) Instead of "cheating," you get to choose. That's a great, healthful eating lesson for anyone.

AMY'S STORY

"I gained weight with my kids, but not from pregnancy. I'm thirty-eight, and I have a four-year-old and work part-time at home as a tax preparer. You know what happens with a kid. You feed them lunch and you eat the leftover chicken nuggets. There's always food in the kitchen, a temptation I didn't have when I worked in an office. My son would be crying, the phone would be ringing, work wasn't getting done, I'd get stressed and I'd eat.

"My doctor warned me that if I didn't start to lose weight now, I could be at risk for a heart attack in the future.

"What I got out of the weight management program for women was a feeling of finally being in control. I learned why I was overeating, how I was using food to comfort myself. Now I throw away the leftovers, and if I want dessert, I know I can have it in exchange for something else. I feel much better about myself, more in control when I know I can make choices. That's the biggest plus. The extra benefit is that as my weight started going down, my blood pressure and my cholesterol went down, too."

SAMPLE MEAL PLANS

	1,200 CALORIES		1,400 CALORIES		1,600 CALORIES
MEAL PLAN	**MENU**	**MEAL PLAN**	**MENU**	**MEAL PLAN**	**MENU**
BREAKFAST					
1 Starch	¾ cup of cereal	1 Starch	¾ cup cereal	2 Starch	2 slices wheat toast
1 Fruit	½ banana	1 Fruit	1 small peach	Fruit	½ cup orange juice
1 Milk	1 cup 1% lowfat milk	1 Milk	1 cup 1% lowfat milk	Milk	1 cup 1% lowfat milk
				2 Fat	2 teaspoons margarine
LUNCH					
2 Starch	2 slices of bread	2 Starch	1 large roll	2 Starch	2 slices rye bread
2 Meat	½ cup of tuna	2 Meat	2 ounces turkey	3 Meat	3 ounces lean roast beef
1 Vegetable	1 cup carrot sticks	1 Vegetable	1 cup raw veggies	1 Vegetable	1 cup raw carrots
½ Fat	1 teaspoon diet mayo	1 Fruit	1 small apple	2 Fruit	1 large apple
		1 Fat	1 teaspoon diet mayo	1 Fat	1 teaspoon mayo
SNACK					
1 Milk	1 cup sugar-free yogurt	1 Milk	1 cup sugar-free yogurt	1 Starch	3 cups plain popcorn (air-popped)
1 Fruit	1 small peach	1 Fruit	½ banana		
DINNER					
2 Starch	1 cup pasta	2 Starch	1 medium potato	1 Starch	⅓ cup sweet potato
3 Meat	3 ounces skinless chicken	3 Meat	3 ounces fish	3 Meat	3 ounces lean pork
2 Vegetable	1 cup steamed broccoli	2 Vegetable	1 cup green beans	2 Vegetable	1 cup collard greens
1 Fat	1 teaspoon margarine	2½ Fat	2½ teaspoons margarine	1 Fat	1 teaspoon margarine
		1 Fruit	1 small orange		
SNACK					
None		None		1 Milk	1 cup 1% lowfat milk
				1 Fruit	1 cup strawberries

Source: NYU Medical Center Health Education Center.

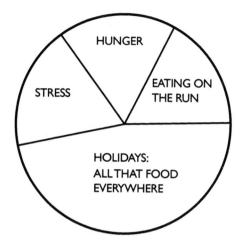

Why are you eating too much?

UNDERSTANDING OVEREATING

The second component of NYU's Weight Management Program for Women has to do with understanding situations that trigger overeating. Stack uses a pie chart to help people analyze some of the reasons they may be eating too much.

This particular pie was carved up during December, the month when many of us seem to put on extra pounds, because of all those fattening holiday goodies and the stress of juggling family, work and holiday obligations.

"People need to start thinking of their weight problem as a collection of individual factors that change from time to time. They constantly need to be evaluating why they are overeating," Stack advises. "For most people, hunger is only a sliver of the pie, but stress, anger, frustration, loneliness, are much bigger portions of the pie. Food distracts us, comforts us, numbs us. Those are the issues that need to be addressed, not just food."

What's the biggest slice of *your* pie? Slice up the pie on this page.

Another useful way to start changing your eating habits is by keeping a food diary. Write down what you eat, when and where you eat it, and why. For example, some people crave afternoon snacks, especially fats and sweets. These provide a quick energy lift. Most people need a snack to

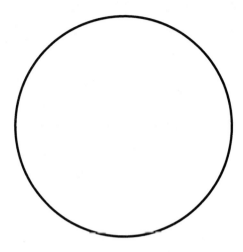

Create your own "pie" chart.
Source: Jennifer Stack, M.S., R.D.

avoid overeating at supper. Just choose healthful snack foods, like fruit or low-fat yogurt.

Many people also snack in front of the television or at their desk. When you're occupied with another activity, you lose track of how much you put into your mouth. So make it a rule never to eat while doing something else, Stack advises.

Other people overeat because they eat too fast. "It takes approximately twenty minutes for your brain to register fullness from your food intake. Give your body enough time to feel full and satisfied, and you'll often eat less as well," she says.

Where you eat is important. Have meals sitting down at the kitchen or dining room table and at a lunchroom at work. Never eat standing up. You know what we mean: a late night nosh standing in front of an open fridge, a couple of cookies from the cookie jar, a "taste" or two (or three) while cooking. These calories seem harmless, but they add up.

Remove temptation from your home and workplace. It's OK to have a weekly indulgence, but buy it in a small, single serving size so there won't be any nibbles left over.

Speaking of nibbles, many women have been raised with the belief that it's a sin to waste food, and they may consume hundreds of extra calories by eating what's left on their kids' plates (as Amy did). If leftovers are a problem, cut back on portions and use leftovers to create another meal.

Be sure to eat breakfast. Running on empty most of the day results in decreased energy and increased hunger at night, setting you up for eating too much in the evening. Also, if you eat too little during the day, psychologically you may feel like you "deserve" a big meal at night. And some studies suggest consuming the majority of a day's calories late in the day makes weight loss more difficult.

TIPS FOR SHOPPING, COOKING AND INDULGING

FOOD SHOPPING

- Never shop on an empty stomach. Plan meals when you're not hungry and make a list of the foods you need at that time.
- Always shop with the list and stick to it.
- Try to shop in stores that stock fresh produce, meat and poultry. Avoid prepackaged foods, snacks and convenience stores. Check food labels for hidden fat.
- If you need only a few items, shop with a basket rather than a cart. Avoid impulse buys; they're usually high in fat.

COOKING

- Try using broth, wine, tomato juice or cooking sprays to sauté foods. Experiment with spices.
- To make less seem like more, cut foods into small pieces. Cook meats and other protein foods with plenty of cut-up vegetables.
- Use lower-fat (or nonfat) alternatives wherever possible.
- To prevent overtasting, while you cook, have a low-calorie snack beforehand.
- Find more healthful ways to cook favorite ethnic dishes.

INDULGING

- Treat yourself to a 200–300-calorie "indulgence" once a week to satisfy your craving for fats or sweets. Your weekly treat might be a small candy bar or piece of cake, a scoop of ice cream, a small fast-food hamburger, or small amount of potato chips or french fries.

• If you want an alcoholic drink when dining out, have a small glass of wine *instead* of a fattening hors d'oeuvre.
• If you want dessert, split it with a companion.
• At family or holiday gatherings, where the emotional or social pressure to eat more than you want is often greater, take little tastes of everything on a smaller plate. That way, you can please the cook without making yourself feel guilty.

THE DIFFERENCE BETWEEN HUNGER AND APPETITE

When you're truly hungry, Stack explains, you have a physical need for food. Your tummy may growl and you may feel empty. On the other hand, appetite is a *psychological* desire for food, not a true *need* for food.

For example, you wander into the kitchen and can't decide what to eat. This may be your appetite acting up. You may need some nonfood solutions to the problem. (For help in recognizing your stress triggers and ways to defuse them, see Chapter 8.)

Parties and restaurants seem to trigger overeating; studies show people eat more when they're in a group. Plan ahead. Consider what you might be eating and how it fits in with your meal plans. At a party, allow yourself moderate portions of special holiday foods and skip the high-fat snacks you can get anytime, like chips and nuts. Eat a low-calorie snack before going to special events. Remember to factor in alcohol (it contains calories and makes you eat more), and don't let anyone (even Mom) push you into eating anything you don't want.

WHEN YOU FALL OFF THE WAGON

The most common hurdle for anyone trying to lose weight is getting over an episode of overindulgence. Stack's advice on what to do:

• Delay eating the tempting food for ten to fifteen minutes; the urge will probably pass. Or delay eating it until you feel more in control of yourself.

- Give yourself a small or moderate portion to quiet the urge but not overload on fat and calories.

- Compensate by eating a little less fat and fewer calories later in the day or on the following day, but don't skip meals.

- Increase your exercise to help burn off the excess calories.

If you really overdo it, stay cool, give yourself a pep talk and quietly dispose of the problem food. Plan sensible ways to compensate for your binge; examine what led you to overeat so you don't repeat the episode. Above all, don't give up on healthful eating!

6

Eating for the Rest of Your Life

IN THE PAST few years, researchers have learned that eating the right foods is one of the best preventive medicines for heart disease (and cancer as well).

Once you know the foods that are good for your heart, it's easier to start eating healthfully.

CUT BACK ON FAT

The American Heart Association and the National Cholesterol Education Program both recommend no more than 30 percent of a day's calories should come from fat. However, many experts now say that fat intake should be no more than 25 to 20 percent of calories, and that more attention should be paid to *the type of fat* eaten.

No more than 10 percent of the day's total fat grams should come from saturated fat (mostly found in animal fat and whole-milk dairy products), which can raise blood cholesterol. The other fat calories should come from healthier monounsaturated and polyunsaturated fats (see page 64).

By switching to this kind of low-fat diet, you may actually decrease your risk of a heart attack almost overnight! Scientists at the Medical

Research Council in London say high-fat meals activate a substance in the blood called Factor VII, which speeds up clotting over six or seven hours.

Since most of us eat our big meal at night (and most heart attacks occur in the early morning), scientists theorize that a high-fat dinner could cause formation of a deadly clot before breakfast. However, low-fat meals quickly deactivate Factor VII.

FIGURING OUT YOUR FAT

To figure out how many grams of fat you should eat per day for a specific level of calorie consumption, multiply your total daily calorie intake by .30 (for 30 percent calories from fat) then divide that total by 9 (there are nine calories in each gram of fat). For diets of 25 or 20 percent of calories from fat, multiply total calories by .25 or .20, then divide by 9. Examples are shown below.

TOTAL CALORIES PER DAY	30% CALORIES FROM FAT	25% CALORIES FROM FAT	20% CALORIES FROM FAT
1,200	40 gm total	33 gm total	26 gm total
1,400	46 gm	38 gm	31 gm
1,600	53 gm	44 gm	35 gm
1,800	60 gm	50 gm	40 gm
2,000	66 gm	55 gm	44 gm
2,200	73 gm	61 gm	48 gm
2,500	83 gm	69 gm	55 gm

Trimming dietary fat can be especially important for women entering the postmenopausal cardiac danger zone, and it's not that difficult to do. A recent study showed that women ages forty-five to sixty-nine were able to successfully cut their fat intake nearly in half *without* extraordinary measures. The study, by the Methodist Hospital and the Baylor College of Medicine in Houston, Texas, followed a group of 303 women for six months, while they learned new ways of eating. The women cut their fat consumption from 39 percent of calories from fat to 20 percent, simply by cutting down on fats, oils and red meats, and substituting low-fat for whole-milk dairy products. The result: They lost an average of 6.2 pounds and their cholesterol dropped as well.

By the way, the *biggest* source of fat in the diets of American women ages nineteen to fifty is not meat. It's salad dressing. The amount of fat in just a quarter of a cup of salad dressing is more than half of what you should eat for the entire day! So when you use vinegar and oil on your salad, go *lightly* on the oil, and be aware of the fat in salad dressings and spreads (again, olive oil is considered the best of the bunch). Next on the list are margarine and cheese, with ground beef coming in at number four. To trim the fat here, see our substitutions list on page 103.

MARIA'S STORY

"I'm over seventy. My generation was brought up to believe the more beef, butter, eggs and milk you ate, the healthier you would be. My husband died suddenly of a heart attack when he was fifty-five. But I never thought about changing the way I cooked until I started having angina myself, seven years ago. I intend to be around for my grandchildren.

"I realized that when my parents had very little money during the depression, we ate much healthier. We were brought up on a mediterranean diet: pasta, different kinds of vegetables, rice, beans, very little meat. We never had rich desserts. The fruit bowl was always out on the table. Now I went back to the old style of cooking I had while growing up.

"My advice to young women today is to avoid sugar, salt and fat, and you'll be OK. Do it now, so you won't have trouble later.

"You can make things taste good without butter and fat and cream. Use a little less oil, just coat the pan. I make omelettes with egg whites and leave in one yolk for the flavor and color. It tastes just as good.

"But you have to stick with it. You can't say, 'I'll eat bacon today, it's only once—I'll have a big piece of meat; it's only once—I'll have the cheesecake, it's only once.' What ends up happening is you're putting that fat in your body every day. According to my doctor, when you eat something really fatty, your cholesterol stays high for forty-eight hours. If you keep eating like that, it will stay up there."

TIPS FOR TRIMMING DIETARY FAT

The Third National Health and Nutrition Examination Survey (NHANES) reported in 1994 that the average American consumes about 34 percent of daily calories in fat. On a diet of 2,000 calories a day, that's about 76 grams of fat. To bring fat intake down to 30 percent of those calories, you'll need to trim just 10 grams of fat a day (see chart on page 101). Here are some easy tips from NYU's Weight Management Program for Women that can help:

SUBSTITUTIONS FOR LOWER FAT INTAKE

INSTEAD OF	TRY
Frying in oil	Sauté in broth
Browning in butter	Cooking spray
Bacon fat	Teaspoon real or imitation bacon bits
Stick margarine	Soft "diet" tub margarine
Sour cream	Plain low-fat yogurt
Ground chuck	Ground turkey breast
Whole milk	Skim milk
Ice cream	Low or nonfat frozen yogurt
Croissant	Pita bread
Oil-packed tuna	Water-packed tuna
Mayonnaise	Light or fat-free mayonnaise
Glazed breakfast pastry	Plain bagel
Sausage pizza	Veggie pizza
Fried chicken	Broiled skinless chicken breast
6 ounces prime rib	3 ounces sliced sirloin

Keep portions of all red meats to about three ounces cooked, roughly the size of a deck of playing cards. Choose meats that have less visible fat, and trim away any excess.

NYU senior nutritionist Jennifer Stack notes that meats graded *prime* are actually higher in fat than the same cuts labeled *choice* or *select*. Unfortunately, it's the marbling or fat in prime beef that gives it its tenderness. Leaner cuts of meat come from the muscular part of the animal and have less fat. Extra-lean cuts can be tenderized by marinades containing acid liquids (good choices are wine, vinegar or citrus fruit juices) by slicing extra thin or by pounding with a meat mallet.

Limit consumption of fatty meats like bacon, sausage, corned beef, goose and domestic duck. Choose sirloin instead of chuck; white-meat turkey or chicken over dark meat; trimmed boneless pork cutlets over spareribs. Three ounces of lean roasted pork has about 11 grams of fat and only 3.8 grams of saturated fat, compared with three ounces of T-bone steak having about 24 grams of fat, 10 of them saturated.

Eat at least two low-fat fish meals a week, such as salmon or tuna, which are rich in polyunsaturated *omega-3 fatty acids*; omega-3s may also help lower your triglycerides, reduce blood pressure and lessen blood clotting (see page 124).

When choosing prepared or packaged foods, look for total grams of fat and saturated fat, not the percentage of fat. New food-labeling laws that took effect in May 1994 should make this task much easier by setting standards for terms like *low fat*.

For example, a typical "serving" of cheese is one ounce, which contains about 100 calories and 9–10 grams of fat. Under the law, a standardized serving of cheese must contain less than 3 grams of fat to be called "low fat." (*Low saturated fat* means 1 gram or less per serving.)

"Light" means the food must have half the fat (and one third or fewer calories) than the food with which it's being compared. So a serving of "light" cheese has to have under 5 grams of fat (and under 67 calories), compared with the full-fat version. To be labeled *reduced* or *less*, a serving would have to contain 25 percent less of those nutrients. "Fat-free" means a food must contain fewer than 0.5 grams of fat per serving.

Think *low-fat ethnic*. Traditional ethnic fare—"Soul Food," Mexican-American, Italian, Mediterranean, Caribbean, Creole and Native-American dishes—contain many heart-healthy foods like beans, greens and grains, but gain extra fat in the preparation. For example, black-eyed peas, okra, turnip greens, red beans and rice are all loaded with vitamins, minerals and fiber. But by adding lard (or fatback), deep frying, "smothering" in butter or cheese toppings, you've added unhealthful amounts of saturated fat.

Many people think it's more expensive and complicated to cook low-fat foods, but it's not true. Use spices, instead of fats, to add flavor. If you need some ideas to help get you started, there's a list of heart-healthy cookbooks in Appendix III (including plenty of ethnic recipes).

HEART AND "SOUL"

According to Keith C. Ferdinand, M.D., former chairman of the Association of Black Cardiologists (ABC), African-American women may meet strong resistance from their families to changes in their diets, because many blacks view healthful foods as "white" foods and prefer their own traditional "black" dishes.

African-American "soul food" is actually southern regional cooking adapted by blacks during slavery. It uses the fatty cuts of pork like chitterlings, fatback and pigs' feet that whites had left to the slaves, notes Waine Kong, Ph.D., executive director of ABC. Animal fats such as bacon grease or lard were used to fry foods and as seasoning for regional vegetables like collard and turnip greens, mustard, kale, spinach, corn and okra. Meats were traditionally preserved in or cured in salt. Higher salt content in other foods evolved in southern cooking partly to guard against fluid loss because of sweating in hot weather.

While no one lives on a steady diet of "soul" foods these days, salt and grease have become a lethal combination in the diets of African Americans, notes Dr. Kong.

You don't have to give up your family's favorite foods, however. Just make some changes in preparation. Eliminate lard and other animal-fat seasonings. For bacon flavor in greens, add a tiny amount of real or imitation crumbled bacon bits. Cut the amount of margarine or shortening in recipes by one fourth. Steam vegetables and top with seasoned onions sautéed with lower nonfat cooking spray. Avoid frying. Instead of salt, try hot sauces and other condiments, which also have fewer calories.

Cultural foods of the African "diaspora" include dishes like yams and squash, as well as other vegetables and grains. Experts say making a diet more "African" than "American" will make it more healthful; intake of fiber in many African countries is often three times greater than the recommended level for Americans.

REDUCE CHOLESTEROL

Limit your daily intake of cholesterol to *under 300* milligrams, and increase your intake of fruits, vegetables, chicken breast (without skin), fish, complex carbohydrates like pasta, and fiber-rich beans and grains.

Beware of labels that make "no cholesterol" claims; some foods have no cholesterol to begin with. By law, a low-cholesterol product is supposed to contain fewer than 20 milligrams of cholesterol per serving and a product that says "no cholesterol" must have less than 2 milligrams per serving.

Many red meats are high in cholesterol (and saturated fat). But you needn't deprive yourself. If you're having sliced London broil for dinner, keep the portion modest and have a low-fat, low-cholesterol lunch like a salad (but watch the oil in the dressing).

Eat eggs less often and try egg-white omelettes instead of those made with a whole egg, since cholesterol lurks in the yolk. Egg substitutes can be used for many recipes to cut down on cholesterol (but try to choose egg substitutes with fewer than 55 calories per half cup), or alternate every other whole egg with two egg whites and you'll still reduce the cholesterol considerably.

Seafood is generally low in cholesterol, but some varieties can have more than meat, including shrimp, crab, oysters, eel and squid (calamari). However, they are low in saturated fat, so they provide a good alternative to red meat.

The good news is that many supermarkets are helping consumers eat more healthfully by listing the fat and cholesterol contents of meats and other fresh foods, or are providing nutritional leaflets for you to refer to while shopping.

Use the fat, calorie and cholesterol chart in Appendix II as a guide for making smart choices for a heart-healthy diet that's lower in saturated fat and cholesterol.

MYRA'S STORY

"It wasn't hard to change my diet after I had a heart attack. That's enough to make you swear off fried chicken forever. I was told to make big changes and I did.

"I learned to make everything fresh. Low fat, low salt. Baked, not fried. I come from a long line of southern cooks, everything fried in oil, even the vegetables. Butter always on the table, on everything, on the grits, on the biscuits. Heavy, heavy food. Big meals. Ribs was our favorite meal before. Not now. I changed the way I cooked overnight. I had to.

"My three sons hated it. They'd complain all the time that I wasn't cooking the way they liked. It was real rough for a while. Sometimes they'd go out to McDonald's instead of eating at home. One night, I was so upset I cried at the table.

"Finally, my husband told them that if they cared about me and their own health, they'd learn some new ways. And I tried cooking more of the things they liked low fat. So we worked it out."

EAT MORE FOODS RICH IN
BETA CAROTENE AND VITAMINS E AND C

New studies suggest foods that contain heart-healthy vitamins called *antioxidants* can reduce your risk of heart disease and stroke. Among them: vitamins E, C and beta carotene, a nutrient the body converts to vitamin A from dietary sources, such as carrots and green leafy vegetables.

Antioxidants block the damaging effects of chemicals called *oxygen free radicals* that form when the body uses oxygen.

When free oxygen reacts with LDL cholesterol, it becomes oxidized, similar to butter becoming rancid. Oxidized LDL in the blood is sucked up by scavenger cells to form *foam cells* that initiate the process of atherosclerosis. It's believed that vitamin E and other antioxidants may prevent that from happening. Recent studies suggest that vitamin E may also slow or even reverse the buildup of fatty plaques.

Free radicals may also damage blood vessel walls. In an attempt to repair that damage, white blood cells, platelets and oxidized LDL start adhering to the injured spot, creating fatty plaques. Antioxidants apparently neutralize the free radicals *before* they can damage artery walls.

The strongest case so far for taking antioxidant nutrients has been made for vitamin E. An update from the Nurses' Health Study found women who took vitamin E supplements for more than two years had a dramatically lower risk of heart disease.

The study (which has surveyed the diet and vitamin use in a "cohort" of 87,245 nurses ages thirty-four to fifty-nine since 1980) found women who consumed the highest amounts of vitamin E, up to 600 International Units (IU) a day, reduced their risk of heart attacks by 41 percent, compared with women who took less than 100 IU a day.

The effects of vitamin E held up even after adjusting for age, smoking, obesity, exercise and other risk factors, and were independent of whether the women took other antioxidants like beta carotene or vitamin C. A related report, which involved 1,795 nurses who had a history of heart attacks or angina or who had been treated for a coronary blockage, found that those who had the most vitamin E in their diets reduced their heart attack risk by 33 percent, compared with those who had the lowest intake.

Research in Canada also indicates vitamin E may even help minimize damage that occurs in heart tissue during medical procedures, such as bypass surgery. Test results were so encouraging, that a water-soluble experimental form of vitamin E is now being developed in Toronto for emergency treatment of heart attack patients.

As for beta carotene, there is some preliminary evidence that it may also help women reduce their heart-disease risk. The Nurses' Health Study found healthy women who ate just a cup a day of carrots (or spinach, apricots or other beta carotene–rich foods) cut their risk of heart attack by 22 percent and their risk of stroke by 40 percent.

Another study conducted by Harvard of almost thirteen hundred elderly Massachusetts men and women found that beta carotene reduced the cardiovascular death rate by 40 to 50 percent, independent of other risk factors for heart disease.

Experts say one reason beta carotene may protect against heart disease is that, in addition to its antioxidant properties, it may also prevent blood platelets from forming dangerous clots (which can also reduce the risk of a thrombic stroke).

Vitamin C (or ascorbic acid), which is also a powerful antioxidant, may help prevent premature death from heart disease.

A report by the U.S. Department of Agriculture's Human Nutrition Research Center on Aging at Tufts University suggests that vitamin C may raise blood levels of HDL cholesterol. Vitamin C may also play a role in keeping blood pressure in check, by preventing free radical damage to the lining of blood vessels, including the cells responsible for constriction and relaxation.

The most striking report on vitamin C came from the University of California at Los Angeles School of Public Health, where researchers looked at the diets of more than eleven thousand men and women over a twenty-year period. The study found a 35 percent lower rate of death from cardiovascular disease among women who consumed plenty of fruits and vegetables containing vitamin C, plus a daily supplement. There was no *specific* dose of vitamin C cited to obtain these protective effects, but as vitamin C intake rose above the recommended daily level of 60 milligrams, there was a steady drop in deaths. The Nurses' Health Study found no heart benefits to vitamin C.

We will need to wait for the results of a number of randomized clinical trials of antioxidants to know for sure if they have heart-saving effects. One of the most important trials will be the Women's Health Study (WHS) at Harvard.

According to Julie E. Buring, Sc.D., principal investigator of the WHS, the trial will randomly assign forty thousand female health professionals to take beta carotene, vitamin E, low doses of aspirin or placebo to see whether these singly or in combination really do reduce the risk of heart disease.

A separate Harvard study, the Women's Antioxidant Trial, will study a group of eight thousand high-risk women. The women, who have all had a prior history of heart attack or stroke, will be given vitamins C, E and beta carotene to see if they reduce the number of subsequent cardiovascular events.

It's important to remember that the evidence we have about antioxidants is still preliminary, and experts are still unsure about the value of taking supplements. No one should start popping mega-doses of *any* vitamin based on this early research.

You may be able to get a large helping of most antioxidants from diet alone. To do this, health experts recommend at least five servings of fruits and vegetables a day, including citrus fruits, yellow and dark-green leafy vegetables, as well as other foods high in antioxidants.

To maximize antioxidant intake from food: Steam fresh vegetables, cook potatoes in their skins and refrigerate prepared juices for no more than two to three days, since vitamins A and C can be lost from food during cooking or storage; bake or broil meats instead of frying, since vitamin A can also be lost in the fat during frying. Vitamin E can also be lost during cooking or processing; store foods in airtight containers. Most ready-to-eat fortified cereals are fortified with vitamins A, C and E.

TAKING ANTIOXIDANTS SAFELY

If you wish to take supplements, you can increase your consumption of antioxidants while staying within safe levels. **However, do not take any sort of vitamin supplement without telling your doctor first.**

Vitamin A/Beta Carotene: At present, experts recommend a daily minimum of vitamin A and beta carotene at about 2.5 milligrams, or 5,000

IU. Some scientists believe you may need at least 5 milligrams, or 10,000 IU, of beta carotene either in supplements or in food, to achieve a protective effect. Whether more is helpful in terms of heart disease is not known.

Vitamin A is fat soluble and may accumulate in body tissues. Taking more than 5 milligrams, or 10,000 IU, of vitamin A daily can be toxic to the liver and nervous system. The only known toxicity from beta carotene is a reversable yellow discoloration of the skin.

Vitamin E: The recommended daily allowance (or RDA) established by the National Academy of Sciences for vitamin E is 10 milligrams or 15 IU (also expressed as 10 "alpha-tocopheral equivalents" or TE, the most potent form of vitamin E). Both the Nurses' Health Study and the Women's Health Study involve supplements of 100–600 IU of vitamin E, much more than you can get from food.

Although the long-term effects of higher doses of vitamin E in humans have not been studied, it appears that vitamin E may be safe in doses up to 1,000 IU a day.

Vitamin C: Experts say a protective dose of vitamin C might be about 200 milligrams per day. The average multivitamin contains 50–100 milligrams of vitamin C, considered a safe level; the RDA is 60 milligrams. Since smokers seem to retain less vitamin C than nonsmokers, it's recommended that smokers take an extra 50–100 milligrams. Do *not* take more than 1,000 milligrams of vitamin C a day. It can cause kidney stones and other adverse effects.

FOODS HIGH IN ANTIOXIDANTS

Note: Vitamin A is expressed as "retinol equivalents." The RDA would be 1,000 RE. In plant foods, 1 RE equals 10 IU; in animal foods, 1 RE equals 3.33 IU of vitamin A. The food content of beta carotene and vitamin E is expressed below in milligrams (mg).

MG/BETA CAROTENE

FRUITS AND VEGETABLES	MILLIGRAMS
Carrots, raw/cooked, ½ cup	6.6
Carrots, canned, ½ cup	5.3
Dandelion leaves, ½ cup	4.3
Cantaloupe, raw, ½ cup	3.5
Spinach, canned, ½ cup	3.5
Mango, raw, ½ medium	2.8
Mango, ½ fruit	2.8
Sweet potato, cooked, ½ cup	2.7
Kale, cooked, ½ cup	2.7
Pumpkin, ½ cup	2.4
Apricots, 10 halves	1.6
Squash, winter, cooked, ½ cup	1.4
Spinach, raw, ½ cup	1.2

VITAMIN C

FRUITS AND JUICES	MILLIGRAMS
Papaya, raw, 1 fruit	188
Fruit, mixed, frozen, 1 cup	187
Cantaloupe, ½	113
Currants, black, ½ cup	101
Strawberries, raw, 1 cup	84
Kiwi fruit, raw, 1	74
Oranges, 1 medium	70
Watermelon, 1 slice	46
Orange juice, can, unsweetened, 4 ounces	44
Orange juice, fresh, 1 orange	43
Grapefruit, raw, ½ fruit	42
Grapefruit sections, can, ½ cup	42
Mandarin orange, canned, ½ cup	42

RE/VITAMIN A

FRUITS AND VEGETABLES (1 RE = 10 IU)	RE
Sweet potato, mashed, ½ cup	2796
Sweet potato, baked, in skin	2182
Carrots, raw, ½ cup	1547
Carrots, canned, ½ cup	1005
Cantaloupe, raw, 1½ fruit	861
Mango, raw, 1 fruit	809
Spinach, fresh, cooked, ½ cup	737
Squash, butternut, cooked, ½ cup	714

VEGETABLES

	MILLIGRAMS
Pepper, red, raw, 1 pepper	141
Pimentos, canned, 4 ounces	107
Pepper, green/red, cooked, 1	81
Sweet potato, canned, ½ cup	53
Broccoli, cooked, ½ cup	49
Broccoli, raw, ½ cup	41
Kale, raw, ½ cup	41
Cauliflower, fresh/raw, ½ cup	36
Peas, raw, ½ cup	31

RE/VITAMIN A

FRUITS AND VEGETABLES (1 RE = 10 IU)	RE
Peas/carrots, cooked, ½ cup	621
Kale, fresh, cooked, ½ cup	481
Sweet red pepper, raw, 1 small	422
Turnip greens, cooked, ½ cup	396
Melon balls, frozen, 1 cup	307

VEGETABLES

	MILLIGRAMS
Sweet potato, cooked, ½ cup	28
Kale, fresh, cooked, ½ cup	27
Asparagus, fresh, cooked, ½ cup	24
Potato, baked w/skin, 1 medium	26
Potato, boiled w/skin, ½ cup	10

MEATS (1 RE = 3.33 IU)	RE
Liver, beef, braised, 3 ounces	9011
Liver, chicken, simmered, 1 cup	6878
Liver, pork, braised, 3 ounces	4589

MG/VITAMIN E

OILS AND NUTS	MILLIGRAMS
Corn oil, 1 teaspoon	11.2
Soybean oil, 1 teaspoon	12.6
Corn oil margarine, 1 tablespoon	9.5
Wheat germ, plain, 1 ounce	8
Safflower oil margarine (tub), 1 tablespoon	6.8
Almonds, blanched, 1 ounce	6
Soybeans, dry, 1 ounce	5.8
Cashews, roasted, 1 ounce	3.1
Peanuts, roasted, 1 ounce	3.1

Sources: U.S. Department of Agriculture and National Cancer Institute.

BOOST CALCIUM, MAGNESIUM AND POTASSIUM

Scientists now know that calcium and magnesium may play a major role in regulating blood pressure by helping the arteries relax and letting blood flow more freely.

A 1992 report from the University of Southern California School of Medicine at Los Angeles found that for every gram of calcium consumed each day, the risk of high blood pressure is lowered an average of 12 percent. The study, one of the largest of its kind, followed the diet and health of 6,634 men and women from 1971 to 1984.

Magnesium is essential for maintaining the health of membranes in smooth muscle tissue, the tissue which controls constriction of blood vessels. Researchers also say a diet low in magnesium may contribute to atherosclerosis, because the mineral also helps regulate certain white blood cells linked to the formation of fatty plaques. A diet low in magnesium allows too many of these cells to be produced.

Potassium-rich foods may help keep blood vessels healthy. Test-tube experiments indicate potassium may hamper production of free radicals that oxidize LDL cholesterol and inhibit the abnormal growth of smooth muscle cells. This occurs in the early stages of atherosclerosis and it blocks platelet activation, leading to blood clots. Potassium may also help lower blood pressure. One study found that eating just an extra 400 milligrams a day, the amount of potassium in a banana or a glass of skim milk, may help reduce stroke risk by 40 percent.

Of course, this is all preliminary research and you can get many of these minerals just from food. Here are current dietary recommendations:

Calcium: Between ages twelve to twenty-four, females need 1,200 milligrams of calcium per day; adult women between ages twenty-five and menopause need 1,000, pregnant and postmenopausal women need 1,500. Experts say people with salt-sensitive hypertension may be helped by consuming calcium, especially African Americans. Check with your doctor.

Magnesium: Women need at least 250 to 400 milligrams of magnesium daily, more during pregnancy.

Potassium: The National Academy of Sciences says daily potassium intake should be between 1,600 and 2,000 milligrams a day.

FOODS HIGH IN CALCIUM

Note: The lower the fat content in dairy products, generally the higher the calcium.

FOOD CHOICES	MILLIGRAMS OF CALCIUM	FOOD CHOICES	MILLIGRAMS OF CALCIUM
DAIRY FOODS		**VEGETABLES/GRAINS**	
2-% low-fat milk, fortified, I cup	352	Collard greens, fresh, cooked, ½ cup	179
Whole milk, I cup	291	Spinach, fresh, cooked, ½ cup	122
Nonfat yogurt, plain, I cup	450	Turnip greens, fresh, cooked, ½ cup	99
Low-fat yogurt, plain, I cup	415	Broccoli, fresh, cooked, ½ cup	89
Parmesan cheese, I ounce	355	Okra, frozen, cooked, ½ cup	88
Romano cheese, I ounce	301	Tums, I tablet	200
Swiss cheese, I ounce	272	Calcium-fortified orange juice, I cup	300
Ice cream, soft serve, ½ cup	118		
Frozen yogurt, plain, I cup	89		
Ice milk, ½ cup	88		

FISH/MEAT SUBSTITUTES

FOOD CHOICES	MILLIGRAMS OF CALCIUM
Tofu, with calcium sulfate, ½ cup	434
Sardines, canned with bones, 3 ounces	371

Sources: U.S. Department of Agriculture and National Dairy Council.

FOODS HIGH IN POTASSIUM

FOOD CHOICES	MILLIGRAMS OF POTASSIUM	FOOD CHOICES	MILLIGRAMS OF POTASSIUM
FRUITS		**VEGETABLES**	
Avocado, Florida, 1 fruit	1,484	Beet greens, cooked, ½ cup	654
Peaches, dried, 10 halves	1,295	Chard, cooked, ½ cup	483
Cantaloupe, raw, ½ fruit	825	Tomato sauce, canned, ½ cup	452
Prune juice, unsweetened, canned, 1 cup	600	Sweet potato/yam, baked or boiled, ½ cup	455
Apricots, dried, 10 halves	482	Spinach, cooked, ½ cup	419
Banana, raw, 1 medium	451	Plantain, cooked, ½ cup	358
		Potato, boiled, with skin, ½ cup	295
		Squash, winter or butternut, cooked, ½ cup	290
MILK, CHEESE AND YOGURT		**DRY BEANS/PEAS/ GRAINS**	
Milk, skim, 1 cup	418	Soybeans, dried, cooked, 1 cup	972
Yogurt, plain/skim milk, 4 ounces	288	Lima beans, dry, cooked, ½ cup	572
		100-% bran cereals, 1 ounce	350
		Black-eyed peas, dried, cooked, ½ cup	344

MEAT, POULTRY, FISH AND SEAFOOD

An average 3-ounce serving of most meat, poultry, fish and seafood contains 25–40% of the RDA of potassium.

Source: U.S. Department of Agriculture.

FOODS HIGH IN MAGNESIUM

FOOD CHOICES	MILLIGRAMS OF MAGNESIUM	FOOD CHOICES	MILLIGRAMS OF MAGNESIUM
VEGETABLES		**BREADS, CEREALS AND OTHER GRAIN PRODUCTS**	
Spinach, fresh, cooked, ½ cup	79	Roman meal, plain, cooked, 1 cup	109
Chard, cooked, ½ cup	76	All-bran cereal, 1 ounce	106
Beans, lima, cooked, ½ cup	63	Wheat germ, plain, 1 ounce	91
Broccoli, cooked, ½ cup	47	Bran buds cereal, 1 ounce	90
Okra, cooked, ½ cup	46		
Squash, acorn, cooked, ½ cup	43		
BEANS/LEGUMES (DRIED)			
Soybeans, green, cooked, ½ cup	54		
Beans, white, black, or brown, dry cooked, ½ cup	52–60		
NUTS AND SEEDS		**MILK/YOGURT**	
Pumpkin or squash seeds, hulled, 1 ounce	152	Milk, skim, 1 cup	36
Watermelon seeds, 1 ounce	146	Yogurt, plain, lowfat, 4 ounces	19.8
Sunflower seeds, hulled, unroasted, 1 ounce	100	**SEAFOOD**	55
Almonds, roasted, dry-roasted, or unroasted, 1 ounce	86	Clams, raw	42
Filberts, or hazelnuts, 1 ounce	85	Scallops, baked/broiled/boiled, 3 ounce	

Source: U.S. Department of Agriculture.

WHAT ABOUT IRON?

Recent research has fueled a debate over whether iron stored by the body may play a role in coronary heart disease. Iron not only acts as a catalyst for oxidation of blood fats, but may also damage heart tissue after a heart attack.

A controversial report from Finland started the debate, reporting that men with higher levels of stored iron in their blood are at greater risk of heart disease. Adult men were found to have two to four times as much stored iron in their blood as premenopausal women, who lose large amounts of iron each month in the hemoglobin of menstrual blood. The theory is that menstruation keeps a premenopausal woman's iron levels low and may help reduce her risk of heart disease. After a woman stops having her periods, iron levels radically increase along with her vulnerability to heart attacks.

So far, the scientific evidence is inconclusive. A 1994 study by the National Institutes of Health, which followed 4,518 men and women from 1971 to 1987, found that elevated iron levels were not related to increased heart risk. A second large-scale study of almost 47,000 men and women in California came to the same conclusion. However, a small study from Norway *did* find a link between higher stored iron levels after menopause and heart attack risk.

For now, experts say women need not worry about taking vitamins with extra iron, or taking iron supplements under a doctor's supervision to prevent anemia. The body closely regulates iron, so heart attacks from excess iron are unlikely, while anemia due to insufficient dietary iron can be a real problem for many women.

LIMIT YOUR SALT INTAKE

The National Heart, Lung and Blood Institute recommends that all healthy people limit sodium intake to under 2,400 milligrams a day (and below 2,000 milligrams for a low-salt diet). That sounds like a lot of salt, until you realize that just a couple of shakes from the saltshaker (a quarter teaspoon) has a whopping 533 milligrams of sodium.

Reducing salt intake may be especially beneficial to older women. As people age, receptors on blood vessels lose some of their ability to help blood vessels relax. One small study from the University of Iowa found that in people who ate a low-salt diet, these age-related changes in blood vessel receptors appeared to be lessened. This study suggests that cutting back on dietary salt may be able to reduce an older woman's risk of hypertension.

Many foods are labled "reduced sodium" these days, but read the label carefully.

LABEL LINGO: SODIUM CONTENT

Here are the terms that govern sodium content under the federal nutrition labeling law.

TERM	SODIUM PER SERVING
Sodium/Salt-free	Less than 0.5 milligrams
Very low sodium	35 milligrams or less
Low sodium	140 milligrams or less
Reduced/"Light"	At least 50% reduction
Unsalted	No salt added during processing

Some tips for scaling down your salt intake:

• Take the saltshaker off the table. Adding table salt to foods that already contain salt can cause your intake to soar.

• Eat fewer prepared foods; 90 percent of prepared foods contain high amounts of sodium. For example, two tablespoons of oil and vinegar contain about 6 milligrams of sodium, compared with the 237 milligrams of sodium in the same two tablespoons of bottled Italian dressing.

• Cut down on salt and high-salt seasonings in cooking. If a recipe calls for a high-salt condiment such as soy sauce or ketchup, don't add more salt. Use seasonings that have little or no salt—like herbs, spices, vinegar or lemon juice.

• Eat more "reduced" or "low" sodium foods. When you eat high-sodium foods, balance them with foods lower in salt. For example, if you have ham for dinner, serve it with unsalted fresh green vegetables rather than canned vegetables, which usually have added salt.

FOODS HIGH IN SODIUM

FOOD CHOICES	MILLIGRAMS OF SODIUM
Cod, dried, salted, I ounce	1,960
Sauerkraut, canned, juice, I cup	1,904
Pickle, dill, I large, 4 inches	1,827
Soup, canned, Manhattan clam chowder, I cup*	1,827
Bouillon, chicken, from cube, I cup*	1,536
Ham, boneless, roasted, 3 ounces	1,177
Soy sauce, regular, I tablespoon	1,029
Tuna, canned, in oil, 3 ounces*	930
Tomato juice, canned/bottled, I cup*	878
Olives, green, 10 olives	827
Broth, canned, beef or chicken, I cup*	780
Pork and beans, canned, I cup**	770
Pretzels, salted, I cup*	756
Bacon, canadian style, 2 slices	719
Sausage, kielbasa, I ounce*	687
Pizza, 12" cheese/regular crust, ¼ pie	673
Turkey cold cuts, 2 slices*	608
Spaghetti sauce, jar, ½ cup*	500
Frankfurter, beef, I*	461
Cheese spread, processed, American, I ounce	461
Pudding, powdered, prepared w/whole milk, ½ cup*	410

* Average sodium content for produce of this type.
** In general, commercial canned vegetables contain an average of 500 milligrams of sodium per cup and should be avoided on a low-salt diet.

Sources: U.S. Department of Agriculture and National Heart, Lung and Blood Institute.

SODIUM IN "SALT SUBSTITUTES"

BRAND NAME	GRAMS PER 1/4 TEASPOON
Morton Nature's Season	350
Morton Lite Salt (with Potassium)	278
McCormick Lemon & Pepper	155
Papa Dash Lite	90
Lawry's Seasoned Lite Salt	89
Lawry's Lemon Pepper	85
Lawry's Garlic Pepper	73
Lawry's Pinch of Herbs	65
McCormick Lite Lemon & Pepper	43
No Salt	5
Lawry's Seasoned Salt-Free	2
McCormick Seasoned Saltless	1
McCormick Saltless	0
Mrs. Dash	0

Sources: U.S. Department of Agriculture and National Heart, Lung and Blood Institute.

INCREASE DIETARY FIBER

Fiber is defined as any part of a plant that we can't digest. There are two types of dietary fiber and each works differently.

Insoluble fiber stays in its original form in the digestive system; for example, the cellulose that gives celery its snap. It provides roughage which keeps food moving through the intestinal tract, and prevents constipation. Foods rich in insoluble fiber include wheat bran and wheat products, brown rice and lentils.

Water-soluble fiber acts almost like a sponge, using the gummy gel it produces in the intestines to soak up fatty acids and other compounds and carry them out of the body. Soluble fiber is found in such foods as oat bran, barley, citrus fruits, carrots and apples. Some foods, especially beans, contain both forms of fiber.

Fiber's main benefits include reducing the risk of colon cancer and keeping cholesterol in check.

Cholesterol is broken down in the liver to form bile acids, which are used in the stomach and small intestine to digest fats. The small intestine then absorbs the bile acids to be used again. Scientists at Philadelphia's Wistar Institute have found soluble fiber *absorbs* these bile acids so that they can't be used again, sending them out of the body along with waste products. This means the liver has to break down more cholesterol to produce more bile acids, leaving less to be sent out into the blood and then end up on artery walls.

Some soluble fibers are fermented by bacteria in the intestine to form so-called *short-chain fatty acids* that interfere with the body's synthesis of fat and cholesterol. Scientists at Purdue University have found some fibers actually attract fats through electrical charges, helping get them out of the body. There's even some evidence fiber helps control blood pressure.

But you *can* overdo it. According to David Kritchevsky, Ph.D., associate director and institute professor at the Wistar Institute in Philadelphia, one of the secondary bile acids produced by the liver (deoxycholic acid) is thought to be a possible cocarcinogen. If too much of this bile acid is taken into the colon by fiber, it could be troublesome. Eating too much fiber may also interfere with the absorption of minerals like calcium and zinc, especially in older people.

Dr. Kritchevsky stresses that a diet very high in soluble fiber is really only recommended for people at high risk of heart disease; it may do very little for people at low risk.

Tips for reducing heart-disease risk through fiber:

• Eat at least 30–35 grams of fiber each day (the average American only eats about 7–10 grams of fiber per day).

• At least a third of your fiber intake should be soluble fiber, including citrus fruits, carrots, dried beans and foods such as oat bran.

• Don't be fooled by fiber fables. A store-bought "bran" muffin doesn't actually contain much bran, but a third of a cup of high-fiber cereal has almost 9 grams of dietary fiber.

• Low calorie doesn't always mean high fiber. Iceberg lettuce is not a good source of fiber. Add some cabbage, celery, carrots, chickpeas, chopped broccoli or cauliflower to your lettuce salad and you'll easily rack up those daily grams of fiber (not to mention the beta carotene and vitamins C and E) needed to keep your heart healthy.

FOODS HIGH IN FIBER

FOOD CHOICES	GRAMS/ DIETARY FIBERS	SOLUBLE	INSOLUBLE
CEREALS AND GRAINS	GRAMS	GRAMS	GRAMS
All-bran cereal, ⅓ cup	8.6	1.4	7.2
Oat bran, cooked, ¾ cup	4.0	2.2	1.8
Shredded wheat, ⅔ cup	3.5	0.5	3.0
Oatmeal, uncooked, ⅓ cup	2.7	1.4	1.3
Corn flakes, 1 cup	0.5	0.1	0.4
Pumpernickel bread	2.7	1.2	1.5
Rye bread	1.8	0.8	1.0
Whole wheat bread	1.5	0.3	1.2
White bread	0.6	0.3	0.3
Bagel	1.4	0.6	0.8
English muffin	1.6	0.4	1.2
Spaghetti, semolina, 1 cup	1.8	0.8	1.0
Popcorn, air-popped, 1 cup	0.7	trace	0.7
Brown rice, boiled, 1 cup	0.5	trace	0.5
White rice, boiled, 1 cup	0.5	trace	0.5
VEGETABLES			
Brussels sprouts, cooked, ½ cup	3.8	2.0	1.8
Broccoli, cooked, ½ cup	2.4	1.2	1.2
Sweet potato, without skin	2.7	1.2	1.5
Cabbage/Green/Red, ½ cup	2.6	1.1	1.5
Peas, cooked, ½ cup	2.4	0.6	1.8
Carrots, cooked, ½ cup	2.0	1.1	0.9
Asparagus, cooked, ½ cup	1.8	0.7	1.1
Corn, cooked, ½ cup	1.6	0.2	1.4
Green beans, cooked, ½ cup	1.6	0.6	1.0
Cauliflower, cooked, ½ cup	1.0	0.4	0.6
Potato, cooked, w/skin, ½ cup	1.5	0.8	0.7

FOOD CHOICES	GRAMS/ DIETARY FIBERS	SOLUBLE	INSOLUBLE
VEGETABLES	GRAMS	GRAMS	GRAMS
Spinach, cooked, ½ cup	1.6	0.5	1.1
Collard greens, cooked, ½ cup	1.6	0.5	1.1
Kale, cooked, ½ cup	1.5	0.5	1.1
BEANS/LEGUMES/DRIED			
Kidney beans, cooked, ½ cup	6.9	2.8	4.1
Navy beans, cooked, ½ cup	6.5	2.2	4.3
Pinto beans, cooked, ½ cup	5.9	1.9	4.0
Lentils, cooked, ½ cup	5.2	0.6	4.6
White beans, cooked, ½ cup	5.0	1.4	3.6
Chickpeas, cooked, ½ cup	4.3	1.3	3.0
Lima beans, canned, ½ cup	4.3	1.1	3.2
Split peas, cooked, ½ cup	3.1	1.1	2.0

Sources: U.S. Department of Agriculture Human Nutrition Information Service; *Plant Fiber in Foods*, James W. Anderson, M.D., 2nd ed. 1990, HCF Nutrition Research Fdn.

CATCH THE LATEST ON FISH OIL

Fish oil, or omega-3 fatty acids, made headlines a few years back because of its cholesterol-lowering abilities. It turns out that fish-oil capsules don't do that much for cholesterol.

But recent research indicates eating two or three servings a week of cold-water fish high in omega-3s (like salmon, halibut, mackerel, sardines and tuna) *may* help slow the process of atherosclerosis and make blood platelets less likely to form clots. However, the oil used to pack tuna does not contain omega-3s, so stick with water-packed tuna.

As for cholesterol, researchers at the Bowman Gray School of Medicine at Wake Forest University in North Carolina recently reported that a diet high in omega-3s appears to alter the composition of LDL, making it less harmful and less likely to accumulate in the body.

Fish-oil capsules may be prescribed for certain individuals, but the American Heart Association says healthy people should stay away from them, especially in large doses. They can cause excessive thinning of the blood, and some products contain a lot of vitamin D, which is toxic in large amounts.

FISH HIGH IN OMEGA-3 FATTY ACIDS

FISH CHOICES (3 1/2 OUNCES RAW)	OMEGA-3/GRAMS
Mackerel, Atlantic	2.6
Mackerel, king	2.2
Trout, lake	2.0
Herring, Pacific	1.8
Tuna, bluefin	1.6
Sablefish	1.5
Salmon, chinook	1.5
Sturgeon, Atlantic	1.5
Tuna, albacore	1.5
Whitefish, lake	1.5

Source: U.S. Department of Agriculture.

THE QUESTION OF ALCOHOL

A number of recent studies, including the Nurses' Health Study, suggest that light to moderate alcohol consumption may protect women against heart disease. It appears that alcohol in moderate amounts increases levels of HDL cholesterol and lowers LDL cholesterol. The beneficial effects of moderate drinking also appear to cancel out alcohol's negative effects on blood pressure. Studies suggest that alcohol acts in several biochemical ways to decrease blood clotting (including lowering levels of fibrinogen, a risk factor for heart disease).

In addition, a study by the University of Pittsburgh says that the amount of alcohol contained in three to six glasses of wine per week may boost low levels of estrogen in postmenopausal women, which in turn may protect against cardiovascular problems. The researchers believe alcohol may stimulate a biochemical process that converts male hormones, or androgens, into estrogen after menopause. Women who drank alcohol had estrogen levels two-thirds higher than those who did not drink. (The benefits did not rise with consumption of more than three to six glasses of wine per week.)

Unfortunately, the same level of drinking that protects the heart may also increase the risk of breast cancer. A 1993 report in the *Journal of the National Cancer Institute* found that two alcoholic drinks per day raised levels of estrogen and other hormones in premenopausal women by 15 to 30 percent.

Alcohol also makes people burn off fat more slowly than usual. One study found a diet that included three ounces of pure alcohol a day (about six beers or six shots of whiskey) was enough to reduce the body's burning of fat by about one third. Any fat that isn't burned up is stored right where we don't want it—in the stomach and hips—a pretty good explanation of why people get "beer bellies."

Heavy drinking raises blood pressure. Federal health officials estimate 5 to 7 percent of all high blood pressure in the United States is related to consuming three or more alcoholic drinks per day. New studies also show that heavy drinking (six or more drinks a day) irritates the heart muscle, causing irregular heartbeats and potentially fatal cardiac arrhythmias.

In addition, what may be "moderate" drinking for a man may *not* be so "moderate" for a woman. For one thing, women face special problems metabolizing alcohol. Since women have a higher percentage of body fat and less body water than men, and since alcohol dissolves more easily in water than fat, alcohol becomes more concentrated in a woman's body. Alcohol also has a more potent effect on older women because of the increase in body fat that goes along with aging.

On top of that, a recent study found that a stomach enzyme that breaks down alcohol in the stomach is four times more active in men than in women. The study showed women break down very little alcohol in the stomach, so more gets into the blood and into the liver. Some studies also suggest Asian Americans and Native Americans may have a lower biological tolerance for alcohol.

All of which means *less* alcohol gets women drunker faster than men and increases their risk of alcohol-related liver disease and other problems.

The Nurses' Health Study defines "moderate" alcohol consumption for women as three to nine drinks per week, or less. One drink would be a twelve-ounce can or bottle of beer, a five-ounce glass of wine or a mixed drink with a one-ounce shot of hard liquor.

Also remember that alcohol is loaded with "empty" calories. A twelve-ounce regular beer has 151 calories; one and a half ounces of hard liquor such as gin, rum or vodka contains 107 calories, and four ounces of white wine will run you 80 calories. So if you want a cocktail before dinner, skip the hors d'oeuvres, don't overdo the main course or dessert, and your heart will thank you.

7

Get Moving

DESPITE ALL YOU'VE been hearing about a "fitness craze," a recent survey found that only 31 percent of American women exercise regularly. It's estimated that as many as 17 percent of women are completely sedentary. And statistics show that the rate of cardiovascular disease is seven to eight times higher in sedentary women compared to those who are physically fit.

Regular exercise helps improve blood circulation so that the heart, lungs and other organs work more effectively together. Exercise can also reduce obesity and the risk of diabetes, two important risk factors in women for cardiovascular disease. Exercise also helps keep cholesterol in check and can lower mildly elevated blood pressure.

The good news is it's much easier (and cheaper) to work exercise into your life than you may think. And experts now say you do *not* need vigorous exercise to help your heart become fit.

WHAT'S HOLDING YOU BACK?

A 1994 survey by the federal Centers for Disease Control and Prevention found that the most common risk factor for heart disease among Americans is lack of proper exercise. In fact, the American Heart Association estimates that up to one third of all adult Americans (thirty-five to fifty million men and women) are at two to four times' greater risk of dying of heart disease *solely* because they're too sedentary.

Most women know that lack of exercise is unhealthful, but they are unable to get over the hurdles that prevent them from becoming more active. One survey found the big excuses for women not exercising include lack of time because of work and family obligations; fear of not performing well or of being ridiculed; concern over costs; and lack of encouragement from family members. Women most at risk for not exercising are young mothers, who have their hands full with small children.

The most sedentary women tend to be overweight, elderly, African American or Latina. These women are less likely to see exercise as something they can or should do, notes Ileana L. Pina, M.D., director of Cardiac Rehabilitation at Temple University in Philadelphia.

"Some women were not raised in homes that encouraged participation in sports or exercise. No one in their peer group exercises—unlike boys, who grow up viewing Olympic athletes or professional sports stars as role models," observes Dr. Pina. Overweight women may be embarrassed about the way they look and wouldn't want anyone to see them in shorts or a sweatsuit. "Other women simply have their hands full with working and taking care of families and see exercise as a luxury, something for wealthy people who have time and money to play tennis or take exercise classes," she adds.

But you *don't* need special athletic abilities or money for health clubs and fancy exercise gear to avoid the health problems associated with a sedentary lifestyle. You'll derive some benefits simply by increasing your activity level over the course of a week. But your heart gets the biggest advantage when you start a regular exercise program.

AEROBIC EXERCISE AND YOUR HEART

There are two kinds of exercise: aerobic (or isotonic) and anaerobic (or isometric). Aerobic exercise strengthens the cardiovascular system; anaerobic exercise strengthens muscles. Together, they contribute to overall fitness, and any given activity or exercise incorporates both to a certain degree.

Anaerobic Exercise: This activity improves muscle tone, strength, flexibility, and the balance of body fat to lean tissue. Calisthenics, free weights and weight machines are considered anaerobic activities, because they usually involve isolated groups of muscles for relatively short and intense periods. Sit-ups may help firm your tummy, but will have little effect on cardiovascular fitness.

Aerobic Exercise: This activity conditions the heart and lungs as well as the muscles. It requires the muscles to utilize oxygen for fuel. Since the muscles need more oxygen, the heart must send out more blood to the body. Aerobic exercise consists of rhythmic activity that uses large muscle groups (or several muscle groups simultaneously) and is maintained for an extended period, such as brisk walking, jogging, swimming, aerobics or cycling. When done regularly, aerobic exercise improves cardiovascular endurance by increasing the ability of the lungs, heart and body to take in, transport and use oxygen efficiently.

With regular aerobic exercise, the heart becomes used to pumping more blood with a single beat and can accomplish the same amount of work with fewer beats per minute, both during activity and when at rest. Regular aerobic exercise also helps boost the muscles' ability to remove oxygen from the blood; the lungs also become more efficient in obtaining oxygen with a single breath. This is partly why sedentary people huff and puff and their muscles feel sore after only a short period of physical exertion.

Exercise may also help prevent dangerous blood clots, warding off heart attacks and strokes, and may keep the arteries from stiffening as we age. Other studies indicate that moderate exercise (especially combined with weight loss) can reduce high blood pressure without the use of medications. In fact, for about 25 percent of people with mild hypertension, physical activity and weight loss by themselves may be enough to lower blood pressure to safe levels.

Weight-bearing exercise like walking has additional benefits for women, helping them to maintain bone mass to stave off osteoporosis in later life.

ALLYCE'S STORY

"I was never a real physical person. We lived in the suburbs when I was growing up and we drove everywhere. My father wasn't the type to play catch in the backyard with his kids.

"I never learned a sport like tennis or anything. I bought a tennis racket when I was a teenager and I liked to practice hitting the ball against the wall at the handball court. But I never had the money for lessons and probably didn't have the ability.

"My best friend and I had our children around the same time and she talked me into going to an aerobics class with her. I felt really stupid and uncoordinated, so I quit after a while. I know I should be exercising, but I never can seem to find the time. I do worry about it because of my mother's heart attack, because there's a family history."

HOW EXERCISE REDUCES
WOMEN'S SPECIAL RISK FACTORS

The biggest plus of exercise for women is that it slows the adverse changes that put women at increased risk for heart disease after menopause.

Exercise and HDL: The Healthy Women Study at the University of Pittsburgh followed 541 women (ages forty-two to fifty) for three years, and found those who exercised regularly had the smallest declines in HDL cholesterol and put on less weight. Even moderate exercise seems to maintain protective HDL levels. Its benefits appeared to be independent of diet or weight-loss regimens.

A 1994 study found exercise also lowered triglycerides (a special heart risk factor for women), while increasing HDL and reducing LDL cholesterol. Other studies have shown that women who exercise have lower systolic and diastolic blood pressures.

Even if you hate formal exercise, there's evidence that simply taking regular hour-long strolls can reduce risk. Researchers at the Institute for Aerobic Research in Dallas divided a group of healthy, but sedentary, premenopausal women into four groups. One group did aerobic walking at 86 percent of their maximum heart rate, another did brisk walking at 67 percent of their maximum heart rate, and another merely strolled along, at 56 percent of their maximum heart rate. The women in these three groups walked about three miles a day five days a week for twenty-four weeks. The fourth group did no exercise at all.

While fitness increased in direct proportion to the walking pace, HDL levels rose the *same* amount whether a woman strolled along for three miles or did "power walking" for the same distance. The researchers say such an increase in HDL alone could cut a woman's risk of heart disease by 18 percent. These recent studies also suggest exercise can reduce stress, another factor in heart disease.

Exercise and Diabetes: In addition to having a family history of the disease, those most likely to develop Type II diabetes, or noninsulin-dependent diabetes, are obese and inactive women, who tend to become insulin resistant as they age. African-American and Native-American women are at particular risk, because they often have a combination of these risk factors.

A 1992 study from the Harvard Medical School confirmed previous findings that exercise not only helps people lose weight, but also counteracts the insulin resistance that leads to diabetes. It also appears to boost the body's ability to use insulin, improving metabolism of sugar into energy. The Harvard researchers say that *vigorous* exercise several times a week can reduce chances of developing Type II diabetes by about *half*!

In addition, exercise and a proper diet may be able to control Type II diabetes without the use of drugs, reducing the risk of stroke, heart and kidney problems.

However, people with diabetes are also more likely to have peripheral vascular disease—damage to smaller blood vessels in the extremities, which restricts blood flow and can cause leg cramps during exercise. Massage can alleviate this problem.

Reducing the Flab Factor: In addition to suffering a decline in HDL after estrogen production stops, women gain fatty tissue and lose muscle in later life. Weight gain can be as much as a pound every year after menopause.

Because exercise helps the body burn fat more efficiently, women lose excess body fat and gain more muscle tissue. Since muscle is more metabolically active than fat, a muscular body burns more calories.

In a study at the University of California at Irvine, women who walked between thirty and sixty minutes a day, seven days a week, achieved about a 10 percent weight loss within six months, *regardless of what they ate.* Daily cycling increased weight loss to 12 percent. That's about ten pounds on average. Another plus: A fitter person burns more fat both during activity *and* at rest.

Almost *any* daily aerobic activity can be an effective fat-burner, if you do it every day. If you couple an increase in activity with a decrease in fat intake, you'll start to lose weight. And once you start paring down and like the way you look and feel, it's an incentive to keep on eating more healthfully and exercising.

MOVE IT AND LOSE IT

Here's how many calories you'll burn per hour during various activities, based on a woman weighing one hundred and forty pounds. If you weigh more, you'll probably burn more calories. If you weigh less, you'll burn slightly fewer calories.

ACTIVITY	CALORIES BURNED PER HOUR
SITTING QUIETLY	80
STANDING QUIETLY	95
LIGHT ACTIVITY Office work Cleaning house Playing golf	240
MODERATE ACTIVITY Walking briskly (3.5 mph) Gardening Bicycling (5.5 mph) Dancing	370
STRENUOUS ACTIVITY Jogging (9 min/mi) Swimming Tennis	580
VERY STRENUOUS ACTIVITY Running (7 min/mi) Racquetball Skiing	740

Source: *The Healthy Heart Handbook for Women*, National Heart, Lung and Blood Institute (NHLBI), 1992.

SANDRA'S STORY

"Before I started with my church walking club, it was hard for me to go a couple of blocks. I'd be huffing and puffing, my legs were swollen and they hurt. Flights of stairs just looked like mountains to me. Sometimes I would take the bus just to go a couple of blocks, it was that much pain and annoyance. The doctor said I was 'borderline diabetic.'

"Now, you would not believe it! I own a fancy pair of sneakers, just like my thirteen-year-old son! I sometimes go walking three, four times a week.

"I had high blood pressure; now it's down near normal. My blood sugar is normal, too. Now I don't feel right if I don't get my exercise.

"Now when I go out, some of the men see me go by in my sneakers and yell, 'Hi, Slim! Lookin' good.' Now I'm not slim, probably never will be, never aim to be. But it sure does feel good!"

SIX STEPS TO GET
YOURSELF MOVING

Experts say you can change a sedentary lifestyle simply by becoming more active on a daily basis. Here are six steps to help you get started:

1. Become more active today. Steven N. Blair, Ph.D., director of epidemiology at the Institute for Aerobics Research in Dallas, points out that becoming more active doesn't necessarily mean "working out." You can climb two flights of stairs instead of taking the elevator each day and can burn over 100 calories a week. Walk instead of taking the bus, park a little farther from work or the store and it will add up. Walking one to two extra miles a day will burn about 700 calories a week. You may be able to burn 350 calories a week just by taking a walk to window shop during your lunch hour a couple of times during the week.

In fact, 1993 exercise recommendations from the Centers for Disease Control and Prevention and the American College of Sports Medicine urge people to try to "accumulate" at least thirty minutes of such moderate exercise over the course of a day, every day of the week. Dr. Blair stresses that activities like gardening and housework are physical activities, too. You'll burn approximately the same 120 calories vigorously vacuuming the floor for thirty minutes as you will taking a one-mile walk at two miles per hour!

2. Choose a physical activity you like. The best physical activity for you depends on your lifestyle, your medical history, and your desire to keep at it. Be creative, try something new. Learn swimming, aerobics or dancing at your local Y. Pick a time of day for exercise that works best for you. Some studies show that people who exercise in the morning find they have more energy during the day and tend to stick with exercise. Once you make a schedule, stick to it. If an exercise session conflicts with a favorite television show, tape the show and watch it later.

3. Take it at your own pace. The best route to cardiovascular fitness is a regular aerobic exercise program. But recent studies indicate the benefits of exercise do *not* significantly increase along with the intensity of the exercise. And always remember to warm up and cool down (see page 136).

4. Make exercise a habit. Once you find an activity you like, set up a routine. Studies show that once someone has exercised regularly for six months, he or she is more likely to stay with it. Don't become discouraged or upset if you skip a day because of illness, work or family obligations; just resume your exercise program as soon as possible.

It also helps to have someone along to encourage you. Ask a friend to join you, or find out what kind of exercise programs are available in your community.

5. Be sensible. Take things one step at a time. You also have to eat properly, get enough sleep, drink plenty of water and maintain your health to be fit. If you are over fifty, have never exercised, have heart disease (or any other health problem) or have had a heart attack, you need to consult your doctor before beginning an exercise program. A woman with undiagnosed heart disease who starts a vigorous exercise program may be risking sudden death.

If you have a physical limitation such as arthritis, local senior citizen centers often offer special exercise programs tailored for older women and people with arthritis.

6. Get your family involved. Women who are busy raising families can incorporate daily physical activity into their lives by involving their children. Walk to the store or school; buy an inexpensive pedometer to show children how far they can go on leg power; throw a frisbee in the backyard; learn to ice skate or rollerblade together. Discover the bicycle as transportation and family recreation. Get lean as you clean or garden together; buy children their own little rakes or brooms. There are also exercises parents can do together with small children. You'll know they're for fitness; the kids will think they're great fun.

Unless you set a good example for your children, they may grow up to be sedentary adults. In addition, make sure your child's school offers strong physical education or sports programs for girls as well as boys.

HOW MUCH EXERCISE DO YOU NEED?

Moderate exercise accumulated over twenty to thirty minutes every day will reduce your risk of heart disease. However, if *cardiovascular fitness* is your goal, the American Heart Association recommends a minimum "dose" of sustained aerobic exercise of thirty to sixty minutes, three times a week. During this period of exercise, you need to bring your heart rate (pulse beats per minute) within a "target heart rate zone" in order to help your heart and lungs become more efficient. This target zone is between 50 and 75 percent of your maximum heart rate, the fastest your heart can beat at a given age. (You can calculate your own target zone by subtracting your age from 220, or use the chart on page 136.)

Exercising *above* 75 percent of your maximum heart rate can be too strenuous unless you're in peak physical condition; exercising *below* that level gives your heart and lungs too little conditioning. If you're older or have never exercised before (if you're at risk for heart disease or have other health problems), your doctor will recommend that you start exercising at a lower target heart rate and work up gradually.

You can measure your heart rate (at exercise or at rest) very simply: Place the tips of your first two fingers on one of your carotid arteries in the neck (found on the left and right sides of your Adam's apple) and count your pulse for ten seconds. Multiply that number by six, and you have your heart rate.

It's important to realize this target heart rate is *not a goal in itself*, but a measurement of the body's response to exercise. It indicates you're getting the most from your workout. *If exercising to your target heart rate seems complicated, or makes exercise feel like a chore instead of a pleasure, skip it. Just get out and get moving; that's what's really important.*

TARGET HEART RATE ZONES

AGE	TARGET HEART RATE ZONE 50%–75%	AVERAGE MAXIMUM HEART RATE 100%
YEARS	BEATS PER MINUTE	BEATS PER MINUTE
20	100–150	200
25	98–146	195
30	95–142	190
35	93–138	185
40	90–135	180
45	88–131	175
50	85–127	170
55	83–123	165
60	80–120	160
65	78–116	155
70	75–113	150

Source: "Exercise and Your Heart," 1990. Copyright © American Heart Association. Reproduced by permission.

Hitting the Target: If you *do* decide to exercise to your target heart rate, you help your heart pump more blood with fewer beats, both during activity and at rest. You're also helping your heart to become much more efficient over the long term. This is why athletes usually have a slower resting pulse than sedentary people, about fifty beats per minute compared with eighty beats per minute for unfit individuals.

Once your heart and lungs are able to send out enough oxygen to meet the body's increased needs during exercise, you can achieve a "steady state" when your body starts to break down fat to use for energy. That's what helps you lose weight.

However, if you work out too hard, beyond your body's ability to use oxygen, you'll become exhausted and out of breath. Find the pace that's right for you. If you're over seventy, consult your physician.

Warm Up/Cool Down: Experts advise a warm-up period that starts sending blood to the needed muscles while increasing breathing and pulse gradually. It also helps limber up your muscles, tendons and connective tissue. A cool-down period after exercise gently stretches body tissues to prevent soreness and cramps and prevent blood from accumulating in the lower extremities when you sit or lie down after exercising.

If walking is your chosen exercise, a warm-up can simply be going at a slower pace for five or ten minutes before starting a brisk stride. A cool-down may involve simply slowing your pace for five to ten minutes.

If you're doing more strenuous exercise, like jogging or cycling (which can be hard on your knees) or swimming, a warm-up and cool-down should also include overall body stretching. This should consist of slow, gentle stretching of all joints and muscle involved in your chosen exercise.

Avoid Overdoing It: If you're just starting a fitness program, start out with a short period of time, say fifteen to twenty minutes (including your warm-up and cool-down), and gradually work your way up to longer periods.

How do you know if you're overdoing it? Experts say you're probably in a safe range if you're able to talk during aerobic exercise; if you can't speak, you're working too hard. If it takes longer than ten to fifteen minutes for your pulse to slow down after exercise, take it easier the next time. Other danger signals during (or right after) exercise include chest pains, dizziness, breathlessness lasting longer than ten minutes, leg cramps, nausea or vomiting, rapid heartbeats (palpitations) and pain in any area of the body.

WALK YOUR WAY TO FITNESS

Walking is one of the best all-around exercises for people at any age or fitness level. It's easy, inexpensive and doesn't require any special gear. Try a brisk thirty-minute walk during a lunch break, or take a morning or evening walk.

Many urban communities, housing complexes and church groups have started up walking programs that provide companionship, police-approved routes and even baby-sitting. You might find such a walking club just around the corner—or start one yourself! Your might consider mall walking, where climate and safety are not concerns. However, mall walking is *not* for window-shopping. Do that before or after your fitness walk!

If you can afford one, you might want to buy a treadmill so you can do your walking anytime, perhaps while listening to your favorite music or watching a television show. There are also inexpensive "stair steppers" or "ski machines" that can be folded up and tucked away in a closet when not in use. (Those much-advertised thigh exercisers will *not* help your heart.)

However, all you really need to get going is a comfortable pair of walking shoes and clothing that's appropriate for the weather (and maybe a cassette player with earphones to make the going fun). Pick shoes that have thick, flexible soles that cushion the entire sole of the foot and absorb shock for the bones and ligaments of the foot.

Mariano J. Rey, M.D., director of NYU's Cardiac Exercise lab and director of the medical center's Cardiac Rehabilitation Program, says you also need to swing your arms while you walk. This benefits your upper body muscles and makes your aerobic workout more complete. Simply close your fists and, with elbows outward, swing your arms alternately in rhythm as you walk along.

Dr. Rey also recommends having some sort of structured program for fitness walking. "You need a program that's doable and that can be easily incorporated into your life. If something's too complicated, people will be intimidated; if it's too unstructured, people won't stick to it."

This may be just the thing: a twelve-week start-up walking program for women designed by the National Heart, Lung and Blood Institute (NHLBI). It's incredibly simple and can be done indoors or out. The only special equipment you'll need is a wristwatch so you can time the warm-up, cool-down and brisk walking segments.

The brisk walking segment can be done to your target heart rate. For maximum benefit, Dr. Rey advises at least three sessions a week. And remember to swing those arms!

WALK IT OFF: A SAMPLE WALKING PROGRAM

WEEK NUMBER	SLOW WALK/ WARM-UP	TARGET ZONE/ BRISK PACE	SLOW WALK/ COOL-DOWN	TOTAL TIME
	MINUTES	MINUTES	MINUTES	MINUTES
1	5	5	5	15
2	5	7	5	17
3	5	9	5	19
4	5	11	5	21
5	5	13	5	23
6	5	15	5	25
7	5	18	5	28
8	5	20	5	30
9	5	23	5	33
10	5	26	5	36
11	5	28	5	38
12	5	30	5	40
AFTER WEEK 12	5	30	5	40

Source: *The Healthy Heart Handbook for Women*, NHLBI, 1992.

Swimming or water aerobics are also great ways to exercise, especially for older women who may have physical problems such as arthritis. Many local Y's offer water-exercise programs. The cushioning effect of water means less stress on bones, joints and muscles. In addition, the resistance of the water is actually equivalent to exercising with weights, which tones and strengthens muscles, especially the legs, arms and back.

JEANNE'S STORY

"Until my doctor recommended I start doing moderate exercise, I never did anything more physical than rose gardening. I didn't come from a generation where many girls played sports. At first, I was afraid exercise would make my angina worse, but he said for my type of angina it could help. He told me to take it slow and not overdo it and stop if I had any symptoms at all.

"Now I go on regular walks, either in the neighborhood or at the mall. I have a friend who walks with me, and that keeps me from making excuses not to go. Actually, I like being more active. It makes me feel like I'm doing something good for myself, not just taking medicine."

WHEN THERE'S A HEART PROBLEM

If you have been diagnosed with cardiovascular disease, before beginning any exercise program, you need a stress test to see how your heart responds to exercise. The test can detect sudden changes in blood pressure, chest pain (angina) and irregular heartbeats, which may occur during exercise and can indicate the presence of heart disease.

Certain heart problems need to be stabilized first with medical treatment before a doctor may give permission for a patient to exercise. These include extreme high blood pressure, cardiac arrhythmias, inflammation of the heart muscle, severe narrowing of the aorta and unstable angina (where chest pains increase in frequency or intensity no matter what the patient's activity level). Some patients may need a medically supervised exercise program.

Cardiac Rehabilitation: Exercise is also a key part of the recovery process after bypass surgery or a heart attack.

The first cardiac rehab exercises are designed to be done in bed or in a chair, such as raising and lowering arms and legs. These help get blood circulating more effectively and prevent blood clots. If a heart attack is not severe, patients are encouraged to get up and walk around within a day or two to prevent muscle weakness and deconditioning.

Patients are then referred to a "phase-one" inpatient exercise rehab program, designed to improve cardiac endurance and aerobic capacity and to help them resume normal, independent living (especially critical for older women who may live alone). Each program is individually tailored, taking into account any other health problems (such as arthritis).

Inpatient cardiac rehabilitation consists of a circuit-training program lasting ten to fourteen days in a specially equipped exercise room where nurses, physical-therapy instructors and physicians carefully monitor a patient's progress. Treadmills and exercise bicycles are used to condition the legs (some with moving handles to provide a workout for the upper body as well); special machines provide exercise for the arms and upper body, consisting of a wheel with handgrips, and stair-steppers, which are especially helpful for people who have stairs at home.

After a patient goes home, a three- to six-week rehab program of limited exercise is carefully designed to increase stamina and confidence. Patients are taught to monitor their pulse and calculate their heart rate.

"People are often terrified to attempt any kind of exercise after a heart attack; they're afraid of getting another heart attack," says Horacio Pineda, M.D., a clinical assistant professor of rehabilitation medicine and codirector of NYU's Cardiac Rehabilitation Program. "Once people become active, they regain their confidence."

Additionally, a patient may be referred to a formal "phase-two" outpatient cardiac rehabilitation program. Women who were active before their heart attack and enjoyed tennis, skiing or other sports will gain the vitality to resume these activities.

A preenrollment physical and exercise stress test is required, along with a review of your medical history. The program should be overseen by a cardiologist and a rehabilitation specialist, with a nurse or doctor on site at all times. Exercise instructors should have a B.A. in physical therapy or a related field (e.g., exercise physiologist) and special training in cardiac rehabilitation, advises Dr. Pineda.

After three months (about thirty-six sessions) in a phase-two program, a cardiac patient may be able to exercise on her own or choose to continue at the facility. Most insurance pays for three months of phase-two cardiac rehabilitation.

LISTEN TO YOUR BODY

If you experience any of the following symptoms during your cardiac rehabilitation exercise program, stop and rest for a few moments, says Dr. Pineda. If your symptoms don't go away after a brief rest, seek prompt medical attention.

• Chest pain, or chest pain that radiates to the arms, back, jaw or ear
• Dizziness or light-headedness
• Shortness of breath
• Excessive fatigue
• Increased or irregular pulse, persisting for more than five minutes after you have stopped exercising
• Nausea, vomiting
• Excessive sweating, feeling cold and clammy

More and more cardiac rehabilitation programs are being tailored just for women. "In the past, women dropped out of cardiac rehab because their own needs were not being met by the programs," admits Dr. Mariano Rey. "Often they are thrown in with a class of six or seven men and they had no one to talk to or relate to. They may get the same sexist comments and attitudes they are exposed to in general society. Exercise programs designed for women can provide comfort, companionship and motivation."

To find out about special exercise programs in your area, contact organizations such as Mended Hearts (see Appendix III) or your local Y. There are many facilities that bill themselves as "cardio-fitness" centers, but do *not* provide on-site medical monitoring. However, these facilities are perfectly fine *after* a medically supervised cardiac rehabilitation program is completed, and for women who want to improve their cardiovascular fitness.

8

Learn to Cope with Stress

STRESS CAN BE a killer, doing its damage as silently as high blood pressure. It has long been known to cause hypertension, but experts are now finding out stress can also cause dangerous heart enlargement and elevated cholesterol levels.

Stress affects all women. The Framingham Heart Study has found *no* difference in heart disease risk between working women and homemakers. There *are* ways to learn how to cope with the stress in your life and reduce its harmful effects. Some methods take only a few minutes a day and can be done anytime, anyplace.

HOW STRESS TAKES ITS TOLL

Experts generally define stress as feeling emotionally or physically threatened and feeling unable to do anything about it.

When we're threatened, a primitive "fight-or-flight" response is triggered in our body. It sends a signal to the brain, which in turn activates the sympathetic nervous system to produce stress hormones such as adrenaline and noradrenaline. These hormones increase heart rate, blood pressure and breathing to send more blood and oxygen to the parts of the body that need it, such as muscles in the arms and legs so we can "flee"

143

the danger. Sugar and fats are released into the blood for quick energy. Once we're out of danger, the nervous system produces hormones like acetylcholine to counteract these effects, and we calm down.

Back in prehistoric days, the fight-or-flight response helped a human to escape a charging saber-toothed tiger. In the twentieth century, however, this same response may be triggered by an angry boss or spouse, a screaming baby, having too much work to do or even a traffic jam that makes us late for an appointment. Our own anger also produces this same physiologic response.

If stress becomes chronic, people may produce abnormal levels of stress hormones. Arteries stiffen from constantly elevated blood pressure; the heart weakens from overexertion. Heart enlargement may also occur.

Healthy artery walls are able to counter the effects of stress. Their inner lining, or endothelium, secretes nitric oxide to expand the arteries so more blood can reach the heart during times of stress.

However, new research from Harvard found that if a person's arteries become diseased, the endothelium produces less nitric oxide during stress, when hormones constrict blood vessels. The nitric oxide produced may also lose its effectiveness.

The result is *ischemia,* decreased blood flow to the heart, often causing chest pains called *angina,* painful muscle spasms indicating the heart isn't getting enough blood. Ischemia may also be without physical symptoms. Scientists have recently found that in cases of mental stress, *silent ischemia* may occur more often than angina. Recent reports also say stress may trigger the release of a blood chemical that makes platelets more likely to form clots.

While stress hormones trigger the release of fat into the bloodstream to provide momentary energy, long-term stress may damage the liver, causing too much fat to be sent out into the blood—fat that eventually ends up on artery walls.

Recent research indicates that women may have a heightened biological response to stress compared to men, producing more of certain stress hormones. The cardiovascular effects of stress may be worse in postmenopausal women. Estrogen is important in regulating blood vessel tone. When women hit menopause, lack of estrogen creates blood vessel instability that results in hot flashes. Recent clinical research at Cedars Sinai Medical Center suggests that postmenopausal women have greater vessel reactivity in response to stress than men. Stress reactions occurred three times more often in the postmenopausal women, compared to younger women and men. Patients with hostile personalities had greater stress reactions.

THE ANGER FACTOR

Studies have shown that chronically hostile or angry people have five times the risk of heart attack as their more placid counterparts. But evidence is now mounting that the way a woman *handles* her anger may be especially important.

Scientists have been talking about a "type A" personality—chronically hostile, harried and competitive—for decades. The clinical connection between hostility and heart disease was first uncovered in the 1980s by Redford B. Williams, M.D., a professor of psychiatry and psychology at Duke University Medical Center in Durham, North Carolina. Dr. Williams and his research team followed a group of 830 men and women for more than twenty years. At age forty, those men and women who had high scores for hostility on personality tests in college turned out to have high levels of the dangerous LDL cholesterol and abnormally low levels of protective HDL.

A 1992 study of seven hundred men and women from Harvard confirmed that those with "type A" personalities had less HDL and more heart attacks than calmer individuals. Even when other risk factors were taken into account like smoking, diabetes, hypertension, overweight and a family history of heart disease, the type As were at 50 percent higher risk of heart attacks, and had lower HDL cholesterol. The author of the study, JoAnn E. Manson, M.D., co-director of Women's Health at Brigham and Women's Hospital, Boston, suggests that type As' higher level of stress triggers more stress hormones, which in turn have a direct effect on lowering HDL.

Dr. Williams speculates that chronically hostile people may also be born with a biochemical defect in their nervous system that keeps them aroused long after other people have cooled down. This may lead to higher rises in blood pressure, which damage the heart and blood vessels; the turbulence of blood surging through the coronary artery may cause microscopic tears in the lining, hastening the formation of atherosclerotic plaque. In addition, scientists at the University of Miami suggest that chronic anger reduces the pumping efficiency of the heart.

However, women are affected by different societal pressures and roles, which may force them to keep a lid on their anger. Women have traditionally been the "peacemakers" in the family, sometimes at the expense of their own feelings. Women have to keep especially cool on the job, where a display of "female" temper can derail a career. As a result, many women get in the habit of swallowing their anger, which a number of new studies suggest can lead to an increased risk of heart attacks.

Mara Julius, Sc.D., a psychosocial epidemiologist at the University of Michigan, has followed almost seven hundred men and women for more than eighteen years, studying how people cope with anger. She reports that women who suppress their anger were three times more likely to die an early death, especially of cardiovascular diseases, than women who expressed their anger. Women in stressful marriages who suppressed their anger had the highest blood pressure readings of all the people in the study. And the combination of chronic stress and suppressed anger was especially deadly for women in the traditional homemaker role, trapped in bad marriages.

In the Framingham Heart Study, women who reported swallowing their anger had the highest rate of first heart attacks. Researchers at Chicago's Rush-Presbyterian-St. Luke's Medical Center also found that those women who kept a lid on their anger after a first heart attack were more likely to suffer a second. The study, which followed a group of eighty-three women ages thirty to sixty-three for ten years, found that the women who died of heart disease were often divorced, lacked a college education and worked at low-paying jobs.

Working-class and poor women, especially women of color, do have a number of special stresses that contribute to anger and anxiety, adds Keith C. Ferdinand, M.D., of the Association of Black Cardiologists. Living in neighborhoods rife with violence, drugs and gangs, and facing the constant worry about the safety of their families can be major sources of stress.

"The impact of racism, low-paying jobs, perhaps even working two jobs to make ends meet, adds another level of stress for women of color. Such stresses can perhaps contribute to smoking, hypertension and other health problems by leading to poor eating habits and lack of attention to healthy lifestyles," says Dr. Ferdinand.

These extra stresses are more often internalized by women of color. According to a 1990 pilot study of 102 black and white women in Alameda County, California, by Nancy Krieger, Ph.D., an epidemiologist now with the Kaiser Foundation Research Institute, the black women were more likely to respond to unfair treatment than white women by accepting it as a "fact of life," and keeping their feelings to themselves. Those black women who reported no experience with racial discrimination actually were four times more likely to have been diagnosed with high blood pressure. Dr. Krieger is now following up on the study.

Whatever the actual stressor, the message for women is clear: Defusing anger by discussing feelings with other people (spouse, family members, friends), rather than lashing out or keeping it all inside, may help keep your heart—and your mind—a lot healthier.

ROSA'S STORY

"I've been a waitress for fourteen years. You wouldn't believe what we have to put up with. You got men who'll make off-color remarks. There are people who make racist remarks. People will order food, then change their minds and send it back. Everyone's in a hurry, specially during lunchtime.

"But you've got to smile, because they're the customers. My boss doesn't want to hear you're having a bad day; you're having problems at home. So I just smile and say, 'No problem, no problem.'

"My doctor said my blood pressure was way too high. He said I was eating too much salt and gaining too much weight. But I tell you, it's the job. It has to be."

WORKING WOMEN, JOB STRESS
AND HEART ATTACKS

In the 1970s, when women started to make their way up the ladder to middle management and executive positions, many experts predicted that job stress would put women at a risk of heart disease similar to their male counterparts.

But that never happened. While women now occupy over 40 percent of managerial positions, data from the Framingham Heart Study paints a portrait of a heart attack–prone working woman as someone feeling trapped in blue-collar or clerical work, married to a man working a blue-collar job, with several children at home, and an insensitive boss at work.

According to Judith LaRosa, R.N., Ph.D., deputy director of the Office of Research on Women's Health at the National Institutes of Health, the female executive is more likely to feel in control of her job and have more support systems such as household help than her sisters on the assembly line or in the steno pool. Heart-disease risk is even greater when that file clerk or waitress has a nonsupportive boss, little chance of changing her job and has to swallow all of her frustrations because of it.

Women still occupy low-wage, low-mobility jobs in greater numbers than men, trapped by a "sticky floor," not a "glass ceiling." Women still earn about 70 percent of what their male counterparts earn. Among the three million women who work in state and local government, a majority have jobs in the lowest-paying categories, with salaries under $20,000 a year.

These findings have prompted experts to look at job stress in a new way. New studies show that people with the most stress at work are those in jobs with high psychological demands (working fast and hard), but who have little or no control over day-to-day decision-making (having little authority and a low skill level).

Thomas Pickering, M.D., associate director of the Cardiovascular and Hypertension Center at New York Hospital-Cornell Medical Center, says this type of job stress triples the risk of high blood pressure and, in some cases, causes dangerous enlargement of the heart muscle.

A WOMAN'S TOTAL WORK LOAD

Women have a special form of work stress that stems from their dual responsibilities on the job *and* at home. Experts call this "total work load." Most women would call it a new twist on the old adage, "A woman's work is never done."

Today, more than half of women with children under three years of age work outside the home, compared with one in four women in 1970. Fully 75 percent of women whose children are under age eighteen now hold outside jobs. While the numbers of women in the workplace may have changed, survey after survey shows that women's traditional role as "caretaker" of the family has not.

Most recently, a survey by the Families and Work Institute found that an overwhelming number of women in two-paycheck families work a "second shift" at home. The 1993 nationwide survey of 3,381 workers found that 71 percent of women are primarily responsible for caring for children, compared with 5 percent of men. The pattern was virtually the same for cooking, cleaning, shopping and paying bills. The only area where men took more responsibility was the traditional male bastion of household repairs. Men took on even *fewer* household chores if their wives were homemakers; single mothers also bore a heavier burden.

With the aging of our population, more women are also likely to be caring for an elderly relative. The survey found 56 percent of women acted as caregivers for an aging relative, compared with 44 percent of men, and women provided twice as much direct care (14.2 hours a week versus 7.5 hours a week), such as bathing, dressing or feeding.

This greater total work load is definitely having an impact on women's blood pressure and, ultimately, on their cardiovascular health. A recent clinical study by researchers at New York Hospital's Cardiovascular and Hypertension Center found that although blood pressure rises in men and women during the day at work, after men arrived home, their blood pressure and stress hormone levels dropped as they "unwound." But the blood pressure of married women with children stayed high as they coped with children and domestic chores all through the evening.

Problems obtaining reliable child-care and parent-friendly working arrangements, such as getting time off to care for a sick child or relative, can also add to a woman's level of stress. Conversely, if a woman is not at peace with her decision to become a full-time homemaker, it can become a major source of stress in her life.

What's clear is that women, both homemakers and women employed outside the home, have to be aggressive in getting spouses to take on a more equal share of household chores, says New York Hospital's Dr. Pickering. Single mothers need to delegate jobs to older children (or, if they can afford it, pay for hired help) to lighten their total work load and ease some of this particular job stress in their lives. Some women may need to push for part-time or flex-time work arrangements to ease the juggling act between work and family. Studies show that women who express satisfaction with their jobs are happier and healthier—and their children are, as well.

KARYN'S STORY

"I've had three different bosses in the past four years since new owners bought out the department store where I work. The last one was really 'the boss from hell.' Nothing I did was right. If I supervised a display, she would rearrange it. If I submitted a report, she would red-pencil it and demand that it be rewritten. She would challenge every decision I made.

"I'd try to talk to my husband. But he was having problems of his own at work; his company was on pretty shaky ground financially. There was no one to complain to at work; I knew word would get back to my boss. I tried to talk to my parents, but they just said, 'Don't make waves; so many people are out of work.' So I just kept on holding it inside.

"Then I started to have chest pains. At first, I thought it was indigestion. My chest would start to ache after lunch, and the pain would sit there like a lump all afternoon and get worse. Sometimes I could feel my heart sort of pounding in my throat after talking to my boss. One night after dinner, it got so bad, my chest and my neck felt burning and tight—I couldn't breathe.

"I finally had my husband take me to the emergency room—It wasn't my heart at all. It was something called 'reflux,' where the stomach acid backs up into the food tube and starts to burn. They told me it can be caused by anxiety and stress. They also found my blood pressure was way, way up, so they put me on a diuretic and beta blockers, which they said would also help the anxiety.

"I wanted to quit my job the next day. But my husband and I decided we really couldn't afford it. So I asked for a transfer to another department. I really loved my job, but it wasn't worth ruining my health."

WARNING SIGNS OF STRESS

Like Karyn, your body will tell you when you're under too much stress. Your heart will pound, you may breathe hard and become flushed from the extra blood supply. According to Reed Moskowitz, M.D., medical director of the Stress Disorders Medical Services at NYU Medical Center, chronic stress triggers other physical symptoms. These include headaches, stomachaches, tight muscles (especially in the back and shoulders), sweaty palms and sleep difficulties. Your hands may tremble, you may get diarrhea, constipation or break out in a rash or hives. You may feel dizzy, light-headed or have heartburn. Recent studies say that people who are under stress are even more likely to catch frequent colds; stress lowers the body's immune responses.

Emotional symptoms include nervousness, anxiety, crying, feeling on edge, becoming angry under pressure. You may also feel drained, powerless, lonely, self-doubting and unhappy. Just about everything upsets you; you think about escaping and you may even have suicidal thoughts.

There are behavioral symptoms of chronic stress as well, things we do without thinking, such as compulsive eating or drinking, teeth grinding or nail biting, chain smoking or drinking to excess. Some people may gamble, continually show up late for work or go on shopping sprees. Others may just anesthetize themselves with television.

Stress can cloud our thinking, sap our creativity, make us forgetful, indecisive and unable to get things done. Chronic stress makes our sense of humor go out the window.

When symptoms such as these occur together and repeatedly, they may be warning signs that the second silent killer—stress—is at work.

MARIE'S STORY

"I was a teacher in New York City for twenty-five years and, believe me, it could get very stressful in the classroom. I recall there was a very bad period there where I was really under pressure, and that's when I started having chest pains.

"At first I said, 'Oh well, it's just stress.' But when it kept happening, I did go to my doctor. I was fifty-two at the time and I was going through menopause. They did an EKG, but found nothing wrong. The doctor said it was probably just menopause, and he suggested that I take tranquilizers.

"But I kept on having chest pains. Thinking back, maybe I should have tried to do something about the stress in my life. I did have a family history of heart problems, but maybe the stress made things worse. Maybe I could have avoided a heart attack. Who knows?

"After my bypass, I read a great deal about meditation, and decided to try it. It really does help when you're upset or feeling very pressured. I don't want to put any added strain on my heart."

HOW DO YOU COPE WITH STRESS?

Dr. Moskowitz points out that some people deal with stress or anger by drinking and smoking too much and being less careful about their diet, all of which can impact on the heart as well as overall health. Such people are also more likely to become depressed over time, which can compound risk factors for heart disease.

A recent study found the negative effects of smoking are more than three times greater in people who are depressed. Depression also doubled LDL's harmful effects and heightened the effects of a chemical involved in clot formation. The study, by scientists in California and Sweden, found depressed people with high LDL cholesterol had twice as much plaque formation in their arteries as people with the same LDL levels who weren't depressed.

Smoking also worsens plaque buildup; heavy drinking can damage the heart. And studies show women may be more likely to turn to cigarettes or alcohol because of depression, stress or suppressed anger, which could lead to increased blood pressure. This may be one reason why the University of Michigan study found women who supressed their anger were more prone to early death from cardiovascular disease than women who expressed their feelings.

STRESS-BUSTING STRATEGIES

In his book *Your Healing Mind*, Dr. Moskowitz points out that learning how to defuse stress and the "hostile heart syndrome" can help your entire cardiovascular system and prevent heart disease.

For example, he says that taking a couple of minutes for some simple deep breathing can provide benefits. When you breathe deeply, more oxygen enters your bloodstream. Your heart rate slows, your blood pressure comes down.

Taking a deep breath means breathing from the diaphragm, not from the upper chest, Dr. Moskowitz emphasizes. Breathing from the diaphragm brings more air into your lungs.

You can train yourself to breathe through the diaphragm by lying down and putting your hand on your belly. When you breathe deeply through the diaphragm, your hand will rise and fall. Count slowly from one to ten as you breathe in, and again as you breathe out. After you've mastered the technique, you can do it sitting at your desk, or in your car or in your kitchen.

Taking the time to concentrate on your breathing during a stressful situation takes your mind off the stress, calms you down and allows you to gain control. And, it's so easy!

The same goes for muscle-relaxation exercises, which can be added to deep breathing. Close your eyes and with each breath, imagine the tension draining away from your head muscles, your neck and so on. This technique is most effective if your are lying down in a quiet place, but you can do it in any setting.

Exercise, such as walking or cycling done on a regular basis, can also help. Other stress-busters include meditation and positive imagery.

According to Herbert Benson, M.D., director of the mind-body institute and chief of behavioral medicine at the New England Deaconess Hospital in Boston, all of these activities counterbalance the fight-or-flight reaction to stress by eliciting a "relaxation response" from the body. This relaxation response lowers your heart rate and blood pressure and slows breathing, calming us down so we can think more clearly.

Activities that help the body relax have two components. First, a mental focusing device such as repeating words, sounds, images or physical activities. Second, using relaxation to help you shake off thoughts that distract or worry you.

Meditation doesn't have to involve anything more exotic than sitting or lying comfortably in a relatively quiet place and letting your mind wander as you try to focus on breathing or muscle relaxation. Once you can, repeat a word or phrase to distract you from stressful thoughts or events. These are called *mantras*.

Dr. Benson says many people repeat a phrase from a prayer, like "Hail Mary" or "Sh'ma Yisroel" (Hear, O Israel) or "Allah O Akbar" (God Is Great). But you can also repeat things like *Relax* or *Stress go away*. Just about any positive, repeated phrase will do. Try it and see.

Guided imagery, as discussed in the next section, takes this process one step further: You use the time while you're relaxed to visualize positive images or even events.

If you combine meditation with exercise, you'll reap both physical and psychological benefits. Thinking positive thoughts as you stride along on the treadmill, visualizing relaxing images (like a warm sun or gentle wind) as you pedal a stationary bike will help you shed stress during your cardiovascular workout.

If you think all of this sounds a bit wacky, realize that these ideas and techniques have been in use for thousands of years, in different forms in different cultures and religions. Think of a Catholic saying the rosary in a quiet, darkened chapel, or a Hindu doing yoga while soothing sitar music plays softly in the background.

There are many tapes and self-help books available to aid you in learning different stress-busting techniques. Enjoy and experiment with different selections.

CREATIVE VISUALIZATION
TO DEFUSE STRESS

At NYU's Cooperative Care Health Education Center, a variety of visualization exercises are taught to help patients cope with stress. Here are three simple exercises developed or adapted by Jane Cooper, C.S.W., M.S.Ed., for NYU that may help change the way you experience your environment and help you feel more peaceful in daily life.

THE CLOTHES HANGER

If you normally change clothes soon after arriving home, this exercise can be useful in changing your thinking.

As you remove your clothing, article by article, imagine that you are hanging up your problems with each garment. As you remove a skirt or blouse, say to yourself, "This piece of clothing represents a problem (such as a difficult boss) and the problem will remain in the closet this evening." As you hang up the garment, visualize your problems with your boss hung up on the hanger. Another piece of clothing can represent a different problem, or one large article, such as a coat, can represent all of your stressful problems from work.

When you do this exercise, if you find that thoughts of work are intruding, don't become frustrated. Each time you catch yourself thinking about work say to yourself, "Return to the hanger where I have put you. I'll deal with you when I'm ready." Visualize your problems being hung up again. If you practice this exercise faithfully, it should become easier to make it through the evening with fewer thoughts about your job. When this happens, you have made strides in regaining control of your thought processes and hanging up stress.

THE BOX

Before you leave work, or on your way home, sit quietly with your eyes closed and imagine a box sitting next to your front door. The box can be any size, shape or color, but it must have a lid.

Now think of any problems or people from work that have been bothering you, and as you think of them, place them in the box. When you have put them all in the box, close the lid and watch yourself go through the front door.

If thoughts about your job come into your mind during the evening, close your eyes and send them back to the box, and shut the lid. If they persist, imagine a lock on the box, and lock those thoughts inside.

Don't be frustrated if those thoughts persist. With practice, they will hopefully diminish, and eventually, you may be able to spend evenings, weekends, and vacations free from thoughts of work, if you so desire.

If you must regularly or occasionally bring work home, put it away during supper, while playing with the children, or when getting ready for sleep. When you are ready to work, imagine the box opening, and the thoughts coming to you. Remain in control; you are the boss of your thoughts.

If you work at home, you can also create a box to deposit stressful thoughts outside the house.

THE MINIVACATION

Close your eyes and, using all of your senses, recreate in your mind a place where you've spent happy times (perhaps a beach, a forest or a lake). Choose a special place where you felt relaxed, happy and safe.

Take the time to recall the:

- *Colors*
- *How your body felt being in that place*
- *Smells*
- *Sounds*

Picture all the details of your special place, and then allow yourself to be there for a while. When you are distracted, gently bring yourself back to the scene by focusing on the details.

FIND MORE "SELF TIME"

Try to create "self time" to focus on yourself instead of on the stress in your life.

For a frazzled homemaker, sending the kids to a friend's house or a movie, dimming the lights and putting on some soft music while you take a warm bath may be just the mental vacation from stress you need.

A trip to the beauty salon can be a good stress buster. Is there anything so soothing as closing your eyes while someone else shampoos your hair? If you don't have the time or the money, ask your spouse or even a good friend to do the shampooing.

Taking a long walk by yourself (or a bike ride or a drive in the country) can help reduce stress. If companionship is what you crave, plan a night out with friends or form a play group for your kids, so you can relax and socialize with other women. Participate in church or synagogue activities. All of these can help reduce day-to-day stress.

POSITIVE THINKING
AS A STRESS-BUSTER

A landmark eight-year study at Stanford University analyzed the personality traits of almost two thousand men and women who'd had one heart attack, to see what traits might lead to their having a second one. Traits that predisposed men to a second heart attack were hostility and anger. In women, the traits were anxiety and fearfulness.

The underlying factor in *both* men and women, however, was low self-esteem and depression. Those who attended behavior-modification groups and changed their attitudes were much less likely to have another heart attack.

One strategy for altering your way of thinking and self-esteem can be adapted from "cognitive therapy." This is a form of short-term therapy first developed by Aaron Beck, M.D., a professor of psychiatry at the University of Pennsylvania. In cognitive therapy, people work with a trained therapist to learn to recognize the self-destructive thoughts that send their stress hormones soaring.

Many patients are told to keep a diary of daily events, writing down what happened, what they thought about it and what the resulting be-havior was.

Patients then analyze how their thinking affected their mood, their actions and the consequences. Step by step, they learn problem-solving strategies to deal with life head-on, instead of losing control, sidestepping problems or suppressing anger.

Keep a thought diary and review it when you're in a relaxed mood, or do it with a close friend or your spouse. Let them give you feedback on the other ways you might have thought or dealt with a situation.

Every time you start falling back into your old habits of thinking and reacting, a red flag should go up and you say to yourself: "Let me think about this and react in a different way."

It may also help to acquire a more positive vocabulary. Make a list of common negative words or phrases you use. Then make a separate list of new ones to replace them with. Every time you start to use one of the negative words on your list, substitute a new one from your positive vocabulary.

Cognitive therapists advise banishing words like *everything, nothing, always, never, stupid, should* and *can't.* For example, think of how stressed you feel when you react to a mishap by saying, "Everything always goes wrong! I can't handle this!" But taking a deep breath and saying, "I *can* handle it," helps you stay in control and avoid the physical symptoms of stress, notes Dr. Moskowitz.

It may be hard to believe, but changing the way we think, stopping to take a deep breath or even taking a walk alone when things get too stressful can actually help protect your heart from damage.

9

If You're on the Pill

A RECENT STATISTICAL analysis by researchers in the Nurses' Health Study of eighteen different research projects on oral contraceptive use found only a very small relative risk for heart attacks among past pill users, compared to women who never took the pill.

But add smoking to the equation, and the danger soars. Studies show a woman smoker taking birth control pills increases her chances of a heart attack by almost 40 percent and her risk of stroke by over 20 percent.

If a woman over forty who has coronary risk factors such as high blood pressure, diabetes, and high cholesterol takes oral contraceptives, her heart-disease risk also jumps. Even among younger, healthy pill users, a small percentage may develop high blood pressure with higher estrogen formulations.

At the same time, there are many benefits to birth control pills besides preventing pregnancy. Only a physician can decide whether or not a woman is a candidate for oral contraceptives.

THE PILL: WHAT IT IS
AND HOW IT WORKS

Birth control pills were first introduced back in 1960, but the way they work has remained the same: interfering with the hormonal signals that stimulate ovulation.

Ovulation is triggered by sex hormones called *gonadotropins*, which originate in the pituitary gland, a pea-size extension of the brain actually located just behind the bridge of the nose. The *hypothalmus* gland at the base of the brain starts the process by signaling the pituitary to secrete *follicle stimulating hormone* (FSH). FSH activates the follicles in the ovary to produce an egg and release estrogen.

Midway through the menstrual cycle, the pituitary produces *luteinizing hormone* (LH), which triggers the release of the mature egg and the production of progesterone by the follicle. Progesterone and estrogen stimulate the lining of the uterine wall to thicken with a blanket of blood vessels in preparation for receiving a fertilized egg. If an embryo is not implanted in the uterus, a woman menstruates, shedding the blood-thickened uterine lining.

Oral contraceptives are man-made versions of estrogen and progesterone, which block production of FSH and LH and prevent the release of an egg by the ovary. The original birth control pills combined doses as high as 150 micrograms of synthetic estrogen (most commonly *ethynyl estradiol*) and up to 10 milligrams of synthetic progesterone (called *progestin*). Today's low-dose pills contain under 35 micrograms of estradiol and less than 1 milligram of progestin, and there are several varieties available.

Combination pills contain both estradiol and progestins taken in the same dose throughout the menstrual cycle. Biphasic and triphasic pills use estrogen in smaller, varying doses during the cycle. Progestin only, or minipills, contain small doses of progestin and are taken daily. Minipills produce a thick cervical mucus, which slows the transport of sperm and egg and, when taken prior to ovulation, may inhibit implantation of a fertilized egg.

HOW THE PILL MAY
AFFECT HEART HEALTH

While estrogens taken after menopause may reduce a woman's heart-disease risk, some doses of synthetic hormones taken to prevent conception during the childbearing years may have the opposite effect, especially if a woman smokes.

The high doses of estrogen in older-formulation birth control pills were found to boost LDL cholesterol, raise blood pressure and make blood platelets stickier, increasing the risk of blood clots that can lead to heart attacks and strokes.

It appears that current low-dose birth control pills have only modest effects on clotting, although a twelve-year Harvard study of 116,432 women ages thirty to fifty-five found that those women on the pill had a three times greater risk of developing potentially life-threatening pulmonary embolisms (blood clots that can form in the leg vein or other veins and become lodged in an artery feeding the lung).

But women on the pill who *smoke* are literally playing with fire as far as heart attacks and strokes are concerned. Tobacco smoke contains chemicals that make blood platelets stickier, and women who smoke also have increased levels of fibrinogen, needed for clot formation. So women smokers (especially those over age thirty-five) who take even low-dose oral contraceptives put themselves at risk of dangerous blood clots. Overall, women who smoke and take birth control pills are up to thirty-nine times more likely to suffer a heart attack and twenty-two times more likely to have a stroke than women who are not on the pill and don't smoke.

During the menstrual cycle, estrogen triggers production of a hormone called *aldosterone,* which promotes salt and water retention by the body and causes increased blood plasma volume. This accounts for the weight gain and bloating experienced by some women on the pill. Higher-dose pills used in the past were linked with hypertension, because the synthetic hormones (especially the progestins, according to one British study) apparently triggered increased plasma volume and resistance in small blood vessels, boosting blood pressure.

Although between 2 and 5 percent of otherwise healthy women taking birth control pills in higher estradiol doses (between 35 and 80 micrograms) have been found to develop high blood pressure, *experts say that lower-dose pills carry little or no risk of high blood pressure.*

As for the effects of the pill on cholesterol, a 1993 update on the Framingham Offspring Study, which is following the daughters of the original participants, found pill use generally had no adverse effects on blood lipids, although higher doses of progestins could lower HDL.

The American Heart Association's 1993 Scientific Statement on Women and Cardiovascular Disease says today's low-dose oral contraceptives may even have a *protective* effect on cholesterol, depending on their formulation. Pills with a higher *estrogenic* action raise HDL and decrease LDL, while slightly increasing triglycerides. Those pills containing progestins that are highly *androgenic* (more likely to promote male characteristics such as acne or hair growth) *may* have the opposite effect, increasing unwanted LDL.

Progestins in this category include levonorgestrel and norethindrone. When a low dose of these progestins is used, its effects are counterbalanced by the estrogen in the pill.

Newer birth control pills containing progestins that have positive effects on cholesterol (desogestrel, norgestimate and gestodene) are recommended by the AHA for women who have other cardiovascular risk factors.

Past research shows medium- and higher-dose pills *can* have a greater effect on cholesterol and other heart-disease risks, especially if a woman is overweight, has a history of hypertension or high cholesterol, diabetes, or a parent who suffered a heart attack before age fifty.

Cecilia Schmidt-Sarosi, M.D., director of Reproductive Endocrinology and Infertility for NYU's Women's Health Service, says that higher-dose birth control pills are *only* prescribed these days when a lower dose is not effective to prevent pregnancy. Dr. Schmidt-Sarosi stresses that women taking oral contraceptives should be on the lowest effective dose. If you are currently taking pills with more than 35 micrograms of estrogen, you should consult your physician.

Some women on the pill may also have less premenstrual syndrome (PMS) bloat and weight gain because hormone levels are more tightly regulated by oral contraceptives with fairly low estrogen levels. Birth control pills can also protect against ovarian cancer and can be used to control endometriosis (growths of uterine cell tissue which occur outside the uterus and often cause painful periods).

Low-dose birth control pills are a safe option for women over forty who do not smoke and who have healthy cholesterol readings. Pills containing 20 micrograms of ethynyl estradiol were actually formulated with the over-forty woman in mind. In the years before menopause, as estrogen production tapers off, these pills can help maintain hormonal levels and possibly protect women against atherosclerosis. They may also alleviate premenopausal symptoms such as hot flashes, reduce the risk of endo-metrial cancer, benign breast disease and ovarian cysts.

However, it should be noted that definitive studies on the effects and safety of low-dose pills in women over age thirty-five have not yet been done. And the effects of the all-progestin minipill have not yet been documented.

So far, studies show no significant changes in blood pressure, lipids, or blood clotting with the implantable contraceptive Norplant. Norplant consists of six capsules implanted in the upper arm which release small daily doses of levonorgestrel over a five-year period.

HEART DANGER SIGNALS FOR PILL USERS

Women who smoke and take oral contraceptives (especially women over age thirty-five) who experience *any* of the following symptoms should stop taking oral contraceptives and contact a physician imme-diately:

• Sudden chest pain, shortness of breath or coughing up blood in sputum are possible signs of a pulmonary embolism (blood clot in the lungs) or coronary thrombosis or an imminent heart attack.

• Sudden weakness, numbness or inability to speak or move a part of the body, blurred vision or blackouts. These are common symptoms of stroke.

• Leg swelling or tenderness. This may indicate thrombophlebitis, a possible blood clot or inflammation in a leg vein.

• Excessive water retention and swelling of the feet. Edema can be a sign of trouble with the body's ability to excrete water and salt, often a potential sign of hypertension.

• Headaches and palpitations. These both can be a sign of potential heart problems related to taking the pill.

WHO SHOULDN'T TAKE THE PILL

The American Heart Association recommends that women who smoke (particularly if they smoke more than ten cigarettes a day) should *not* use oral contraceptives, as well as women over thirty-five who have other cardiovascular risk factors (such as obesity, high blood pressure and a family history of heart disease). Women diagnosed with coronary disease should avoid oral contraceptives.

In some cases, high blood pressure and diabetes in *younger* women need not prevent them from taking low-dose pills, *if* their disease is being kept under control and their doctor approves, says Dr. Schmidt-Sarosi. The AHA recommends oral contraceptives which lower LDL and raise HDL for women with high-risk blood lipid profiles.

Other experts suggest that women who have had breast, uterine or liver cancer should also avoid the pill. Since the pill is protective against ovarian cancer, women with a family history of ovarian cancer can safely take oral contraceptives.

IF YOU DECIDE
TO TAKE THE PILL

If you're thinking of taking the pill, Dr. Schmidt-Sarosi recommends discussing it with your doctor first and getting a complete physical, including a total lipid blood profile and a blood pressure check.

Your doctor should start you on the lowest-dose pill for three months, then have you come back for a physical exam. He or she should recheck your blood pressure and examine you for edema (swelling of the feet or weight gain) due to excessive water retention. Women on the pill are strongly advised to visit a doctor every six months or so for rechecks of blood pressure and blood lipids.

10

Menopause and Estrogen Replacement

A WOMAN IS at greatest risk for heart disease after the natural decline in estrogen that occurs in menopause.

Estrogen appears to protect women from heart disease by maintaining healthy levels of HDL, the so-called "good" cholesterol, and helping keep "bad" LDL cholesterol low. Estrogen may also help protect a woman's arteries from plaque buildup and lower her risk of high blood pressure and stroke.

However, replacement hormones are not for every woman, nor are they a "magic bullet" that will banish other risk factors.

HOW ESTROGEN HELPS
A WOMAN'S HEART

Menopause (sometimes called the *climacteric*) is actually a gradual process during which a woman's ovaries stop producing eggs and taper off their production of estrogen and progesterone. This process can last as long as ten years before menstruation actually ceases, and can begin between the ages of thirty-eight and forty-eight. The average age of menopause in America is about fifty-one, although if your mother had an early menopause, you may, too.

Once estrogen production ceases, a woman's risk of developing coronary artery disease increases between two- and threefold. For a woman who experiences premature menopause (before age forty, as about 8 percent of women do) or who has had her ovaries removed, that risk increases threefold.

Scientists believe that estrogen acts in several ways to protect the cardiovascular system. As you may recall from Chapter 4, HDL helps transport excess cholesterol out of the blood to the liver where it can be excreted. LDL cholesterol is removed from the bloodstream by receptors found on just about every cell. It's believed estrogen may increase the number of active LDL receptors, especially in the liver.

Recent research indicates that estrogen may help prevent the harmful oxidation of LDL cholesterol that leads to the buildup of fatty plaques.

Naturally occurring estrogen may also stimulate the activity of the enzyme lipoprotein lipase, critical for removing triglycerides from the blood and helping prevent fatty deposits from accumulating inside artery walls. Smooth-muscle cells in blood vessel walls contain estrogen receptors. A preliminary study by Tufts University published in 1994 suggests that if these receptors are absent or ineffective, preventing estrogen from entering the cells, it *may* lead to overgrowth of smooth-muscle cells, a critical step in atherosclerosis.

Estrogen may also prevent hypertension by keeping those smooth muscle cells flexible, so they can properly dilate to accommodate blood flow, as well as help maintain production of the body's own natural vasodilator in the endothelial cells lining blood vessels.

Recent studies also suggest that another hormone, *prostaglandin*, secreted by the uterus, may play some role in protecting women from heart disease (which may explain why a woman's heart risk goes up after hysterectomy).

WHAT IS HORMONE-REPLACEMENT THERAPY?

Doctors have been giving women replacement estrogen after menopause for more than thirty years.

At first, estrogen replacement therapy (ERT) was given in extremely high doses. But in 1975, it was found that those women were four to eight times more likely to develop cancer of the endometrium or lining of the uterus. Taking *unopposed* estrogen caused a natural buildup of cells that line the uterus. Without progesterone to trigger the shedding of the lining every month, these accumulated cells have the potential for malignancy. Use of estrogen combined with progestin has eliminated that risk. Experts now agree that unless a woman has had her uterus removed, she should take this combined *hormone-replacement therapy* (HRT). Two forms of estrogen are used: synthetic *estradiol* (Estrace) and *conjuated* estrogen (Premarin), which is extracted from the urine of pregnant mares. A number of synthetic progestins are used (including Provera). (A "natural" progesterone, identical to what the body makes, is also available for women who cannot tolerate progestins.)

Adding progestin to hormone therapy does produce side effects, including menstrual bleeding similar to regular periods and PMS-type symptoms (bloating, tender breasts and depression). However, the bleeding may cease after a few years.

Hormone-replacement therapy is now given either in pill form, transdermal patches or in the form of a vaginal cream.

In oral form, HRT is absorbed through the digestive tract and processed in the liver before entering the bloodstream. In the liver, oral estrogen helps to reduce LDL cholesterol while increasing HDL. Since hormones from transdermal patches are absorbed through the skin, they enter the bloodstream directly, bypassing the liver; its actual effects on cholesterol are unclear. Women with liver problems can safely take transdermal HRT. Oral estrogen tends to thicken and concentrate bile produced by the liver, leading to gallstones in some women, another advantage to using transdermal patches.

Transdermal patches (Estraderm vivelle) look very much like a round Band-Aid and contain replacement hormones within a membrane that allows a controlled amount to be absorbed through the skin. They are worn on the lower abdomen, the upper thigh or the buttocks and are changed twice a week, although some doctors may prescribe them on a cyclic basis. A minor side effect may be skin irritation from the adhesive.

With oral HRT, estrogens can be given every day or in cycles of three weeks on and one week off. Estrogen can be supplemented by progesterone on a daily basis, using low or graduated doses, or in a larger dose for ten to thirteen days a month. The minimum dose of conjugated estrogen available is 0.3 milligrams, but it is most commonly prescribed in 0.625 milligrams; progesterone doses range from 2.5 to 10 milligrams. Doses in the patch can be somewhat higher.

Some physicians have started patients on hormone replacement when menstrual periods become erratic to alleviate any hot flashes and other symptoms, to prevent a drop in HDL and, theoretically, to conserve existing progesterone and estrogen. However, Lila E. Nachtigall, M.D., an associate professor of obstetrics and gynecology at NYU Medical Center, a noted reproductive endocrinologist and coauthor of the menopause handbook *Estrogen*, strongly advises against this practice.

Since menopause is considered to be the absence of menstrual periods for twelve months, a woman who still has periods (however irregular) but is having menopausal symptoms is considered to be in *premenopause*. Dr. Nachtigall says a woman who still menstruates, although not regularly, is still producing estrogen and additional amounts can be dangerous, contributing to endometrial hyperplasia, a buildup of cells lining the uterus that could eventually lead to cancer.

The only way to make sure you're in menopause is to take a test for follicle-stimulating hormone (FSH), which becomes elevated after the ovaries stop producing estrogen and progesterone. Blood levels of estrogen can also be tested.

The newest wrinkle in HRT is the addition of very small doses of the male hormone testosterone. A woman's ovaries and adrenal glands produce small amounts of male hormones, or *androgens*, which also taper off with menopause. Testosterone increases libido, and the tiny doses added to HRT (1–1.5 milligrams) not only may help a woman's sex drive, but may also eliminate the breast tenderness experienced by some women taking estrogen. Dr. Nachtigall says there is no evidence as yet that adding small amounts of testosterone affects blood fats.

Estrogen cream (such as Dienestrol and Estrace) applied to the vaginal area twice a week combats the dryness and thinning of the vaginal lining that makes sex uncomfortable for some postmenopausal women, and may reduce urinary tract infections. It does *not* protect against heart disease. However, some of the estrogen in the cream *is* absorbed into the bloodstream, especially at first. Some women may need to take progesterone for ten to twelve days a month to prevent buildup of cells in the uterine lining.

WHAT THE LATEST STUDIES SAY

A number of recent studies show that estrogen replacement begun at the start of menopause helps reduce a woman's overall heart risk by one third to one half. Most were observational studies, and experts say the results may be somewhat skewed, because women who elect estrogen therapy may be healthier and take better care of themselves.

The largest observations study to date, the Nurses' Health Study (which has followed a cohort of 48,470 postmenopausal nurses for more than a decade) found that women who took oral estrogen since the onset of menopause cut their heart-disease risk by 44 percent and were less likely to die of cardiovascular disease; there was no appreciable decrease in the risk of stroke. Interestingly, researchers did find a slightly increased heart-disease risk in those women taking *more* than 1.25 milligrams of oral estrogen daily.

Another large observational study, the Atherosclerosis Risk in Communities (ARIC) Study, followed 4,958 women in four communities for three years, comparing the lipid profiles of those who took estrogen with those who did not. The ARIC study reported in 1993 that women using ERT had significantly higher levels of HDL, lower levels of LDL, Lp(a) and fibrinogen (the blood-clotting element that can predict risk of heart attack and stroke), as well as lower blood sugar and insulin. Taken together, these changes could translate into a 42 percent reduction in risk. The study also suggested that taking both progesterone and estrogen appeared to be just as good for the heart as estrogen alone.

But the question remained: Would adding progesterone blunt these apparent protective effects of oral estrogen?

Preliminary results of the first major randomized clinical trial of hormone replacement—the Post-Menopausal Estrogen and Progestin Intervention (PEPI) Trial—show significant benefits for ERT and a somewhat lesser effect for HRT.

The PEPI Trial compared four hormone regimens with placebo: unopposed ERT, daily estrogen with progestin (Premarin and Provera); estrogen and a higher dose of progestin for twelve days of the month; and daily estrogen with "micronized" progesterone, a finely ground natural progesterone derived from soybeans and other sources, widely used in Scandinavia. Researchers followed 875 women aged forty-five to sixty-four (about a third of whom had had a hysterectomy) over a three-year period, giving them periodic lipid profiles, tests for blood pressure, insulin and fibrinogen (as well as mammograms, bone density scans and uterine biopsies).

The first PEPI data, presented to the American Heart Association's Scientific Sessions in November 1994, showed that all of the hormone regimens were very effective in lowering LDL cholesterol (about 14 to 15 milligrams per deciliter of blood) and preventing the elevations in fibrinogen that accompany aging. Both of these effects could significantly reduce a woman's heart risk. None of the hormone regimens appeared to increase blood pressure or affect insulin.

The effects on HDL varied. Increases in HDL cholesterol were highest among women taking unopposed estrogen (close to 5 mg/dl) and that alone could lower a woman's heart risk by as much as 25 percent, said study co-author Elizabeth L. Barrett-Connor, M.D., professor and chair of the Department of Family and Preventive Medicine at the University of California, San Diego. The traditional estrogen-progestin regimens were about half as effective as estrogen alone, but that was still a major benefit compared to taking no hormones at all, stressed Dr. Barrett-Connor.

Interestingly, the micronized progesterone boosted HDL almost as well as estrogen alone, indicating the drug may be more beneficial for women than progestins. The long-term effects of micronized progesterone have not been studied in this country and more tests should now be done, she added. While all of the regimens slightly increased triglycerides, it appeared to be a type that is not harmful.

As for the other cardio-protective effects of estrogen, an earlier randomized trial suggests that replacement estrogen may reduce the number of fatty lesions in the arteries of postmenopausal women. The 1992 study of ninety postmenopausal women found evidence of coronary artery blockages in only 22 percent of the women taking ERT, while blockages were found in 68 percent of those not taking replacement hormones. The Cardiovascular Heart Study examined almost three thousand women ages sixty-five and older over a two-year period and found that those who took estrogen had less atherosclerosis in the carotid arteries supplying the brain (along with lower LDL and higher HDL).

New research also indicates estrogen may help keep blood vessels supple and improve blood flow. Very preliminary studies at the Cardiovascular Center at New York Hospital-Cornell Medical Center and elsewhere suggests that low-dose conjugated estrogens (such as Premarin) given to post-menopausal women may act as a vasodilator, helping to reduce blood pressure. Jean Sealy, Sc.D., a research professor of medicine at the Cornell University Medical College, New York, and Phyllis August, M.D., an associate professor of medicine and obstetrics and gynecology at Cornell Medical College, speculate that estrogens in doses close to the level naturally produced before menopause may help blood vessels keep producing effective levels of nitric oxide, the body's own naturally occurring vasodilator.

Indeed, a small, two-year randomized study at the University of Pittsburgh found that nitric oxide production increased over time in women who received ERT, with no increase in those who received a placebo. Other tests found direct infusions of estrogen dilated blood vessels.

For a very few susceptible women, however, taking oral estrogen triggers the release of renin, an enzyme from the kidneys, which in turn releases angiotensin in the blood. This constricts blood vessels and can lead to a rise in blood pressure. It is not known if using the transdermal patch or a vaginal cream would produce this effect on the kidneys.

Estrogen may also benefit women who already have cardiovascular disease. Scientists at the University of Tennessee Medical Center in Memphis report that estrogen increased the survival rate of women with mild to moderate and even severe coronary artery disease by an average of five to ten years.

Among otherwise healthy women, those taking estrogen replacement also appear to live longer. A study that followed eighty-eight hundred women in a California retirement community found that women taking estrogen for less than fifteen years had a 20 percent lower death rate from all causes than women who did not. Among those who took estrogen for fifteen years, the death rate was 40 percent lower. (Women taking estrogen were also 40 percent less likely to die of a heart attack and had a 50 percent lower risk of stroke.) This protective effect in HDL did not occur in women smokers or women who had menopause after age fifty-five.

HELEN'S STORY

"I think where there's room for more study is how fast the hormonal protection goes after menopause, and what we need to do about it. If someone had told me, maybe I'd have done more to protect myself.

"One thing I did do was eat right. My doctor told me if I hadn't been eating healthy all these years, I would have had a heart attack years earlier. No one ever advised me to take estrogen. I'm sixty-six, and I never questioned my doctor about taking estrogen and he never asked.

"I know women like to take estrogen because it keeps them looking younger, but I never felt I needed it. I had a pretty easy menopause.

"But looking back, my gynecologist knew I had a family history of heart attacks. And they say women who take estrogen are more protected against heart disease, so maybe I should have had it. But he never recommended it."

WHAT WE STILL DON'T KNOW

Despite these numerous studies, and almost a half-century of estrogen use, there's still a great deal we don't know about hormones and the female heart.

For one thing, none of the randomized clinical trials have lasted long enough to determine the long-term effects of estrogen, or estrogen and progesterone, on a woman's risk of developing heart disease. While the PEPI Trial was an important one, it was designed to look at the effects of hormones on biological markers like increases in HDL cholesterol, which could *translate* into a reduction in risk, not at whether women *actually* had less heart attacks or strokes as a result of taking HRT.

Most of the women in previous studies of estrogen replacement took oral estrogens, and it's still unclear whether patches have the same protective effects on HDL cholesterol. So far, the patch does appear to lower LDL cholesterol, says Dr. Barrett-Conner.

The possible negative effects of HRT are also unknown. Many of the women in the PEPI Trial will be followed for an additional three years to determine whether there were any adverse complications from the various hormone regimens. There was a 33 percent rise in abnormalities of the uterine lining among the women who took unopposed estrogen; these women had to switch to other regimens.

The PEPI Trial also found no effects on the participants' blood pressure from any of the hormone regimens. And since trials of estrogen's effects on vasodilation were very small, and very preliminary, data on the actual, long-term effects of hormones on the risk of hypertension will be some time in coming.

We will have to wait for the results of the Women's Health Initiative (WHI) to find out whether hormone replacement can prevent coronary heart disease over the long haul. More than 60,000 women aged fifty to seventy-nine will take part in the randomized clinical trial component of the WHI. One arm of that trial will evaluate the effects of HRT over a period of nine years. Recruitment began in 1993; results may not be available until the year 2006 or later.

A clinical trial is also under way to see if HRT will slow or stop the clinical progress of heart disease in women.

The randomized double-blind clinical trial is now being conducted at fourteen centers around the country. The Heart and Estrogen-Progestin

Replacement Study (HERS) involves twenty-three hundred postmenopausal women with coronary artery disease. HERS will take five and a
half years and will compare the rate of heart attacks, coronary-related
deaths and interventions (like a bypass) in women taking estrogen and
progesterone to those taking a placebo.

ERT AND BREAST CANCER

Also uncertain: Will a woman who takes replacement estrogen be at
greater risk of breast cancer?

More than forty studies of estrogen therapy and breast cancer have
been conducted in the United States and abroad, but the data is incon-
sistent, and only a few studies have looked at the combination of estrogen
and progesterone.

The latest data comes from the ongoing Nurses' Health Study. The
unpublished data, reported in 1994 to the American Association for the
Advancement of Science, suggests that women who use estrogen replacement for five years or more may face as much as a 40 percent increase in
breast cancer risk. However, there was *no* increase in risk among women
who used estrogen (or estrogen and progesterone) for less than five years.
The increased risk was greater among women age fifty-five and older who
had used, or are using, hormone replacement. Past users of oral contraceptives who began ERT had the same relative risk of breast cancer as
women who used postmenopausal hormones but never took birth control
pills.

Some health experts challenged the Harvard figures as too high, saying
five years of ERT use is not long enough to impact that greatly on risk.
Others point out that only 10 percent of women even stay on ERT for
more than five years.

At the same time, a report published in the *Journal of the American
Medical Association* (*JAMA*) in 1994, which reviewed two dozen previous
studies and three "meta analyses" (which pool data from other studies),
concluded that there is no consistent evidence showing increased risk of
breast cancer among women who have ever used ERT.

Previous studies have differed on the *degree* of risk. A 1992 meta
analysis pooled data from studies dating back to 1970 on both estrogen
and estrogen and progestin therapy and estimated the relative risk of
breast cancer was 25 percent higher among women who used long-term

hormone replacement of either type, compared to those who did not (that's a twofold increase in risk). A similar meta-analysis in 1991 by the federal Centers for Disease Control and Prevention (CDC) pooled statistics on the length of estrogen use, and found the risk of breast cancer increased after five years of ERT, going up to 30 percent after fifteen years of use. The risk was greatest among women with a family history of breast cancer and among younger women who began estrogen use before menopause (after having their ovaries removed, for example). However, many of the women in these studies began taking ERT when doses were considerably larger than those prescribed today.

On the other hand, the CDC's Cancer and Steroid Hormone (CASH) study, of eighty-two hundred women at eight sites around the country (the largest population-based study to date), found *no* appreciable risk of breast cancer for women taking ERT (or birth control pills) even after twenty years of use.

Over half of all breast cancers are what's known as estrogen-receptor positive. That is, the tumor cells have receptors on them that pull in estrogen and use it as a growth factor. Many experts believe that ERT itself does not increase a woman's risk of developing breast cancer but *may* promote or accelerate development of a breast cancer that was already present during the early years of ERT use. Thus, experts have not prescribed postmenopausal hormones for women with a family history of breast cancer, and strongly advise women who have had previous breast cancers against taking hormone replacement. However, the 1994 *JAMA* report suggested that the benefits of estrogen may outweigh the risks for many breast cancer survivors.

That premise is being tested in a randomized clinical trial of estrogen therapy at the M. D. Anderson Cancer Center in Houston. The trial will monitor the effects of ERT on volunteers who have been treated for early-stage estrogen receptor-negative breast cancers and who have been cancer-free for at least two years (ten years if the tumor's estrogen-receptor status is not known). The women will be monitored frequently to make sure there is no sign of cancer recurrence and will be tested at various intervals for estrogen, cholesterol and bone-density levels. They will also receive annual EKGs and Pap smears.

SHOULD YOU TAKE
REPLACEMENT HORMONES?

The decision as to whether or not to take HRT is an individual one, based on each woman's own health history and if the benefits will outweigh the risks for *her*.

A recent risk-benefit analysis, published in the journal *Obstetrics & Gynecology* in 1994, concluded that—for most healthy women—the health benefits appear to outweigh the risks of long-term ERT. Looking at the expected health outcomes among a hypothetical cohort of twenty thousand women (half using ERT), the study estimates women using estrogen for twenty-five years or more would experience 21 percent more deaths from breast cancer but would also have about 50 percent *fewer* deaths from heart disease and hip fractures.

New guidelines issued by the American College of Physicians for counseling postmenopausal women on estrogen recommend:

• All women, regardless of race, should consider preventive hormone therapy.

• Women who have had their uterus and ovaries removed are likely to benefit from estrogen therapy. There is no reason to add a progestin to the hormone regimen in such women.

• Women who have coronary heart disease (or who are at increased risk) are likely to benefit. If such women still have their uterus, progestin should be added unless careful endometrial monitoring is performed.

• The risks of hormone-replacement therapy may outweigh its benefits for women who are at increased risk of breast cancer.

• Maximum benefits for reducing heart disease and osteoporosis are more likely to be achieved with long-term therapy (ten to twenty years). Beginning treatment in older women may be beneficial.

• Because of cancer risks, duration of therapy should be minimized in women treated only for menopausal symptoms.

Experts agree that women who should avoid postmenopausal estrogens include women who have a strong family history of breast cancer, a past estrogen-dependent breast cancer or who have had uterine cancer. Women with blood-clotting disorders, thrombophlebitis (blood clots in the leg), high blood pressure or gallbladder disease should avoid replacement estrogen, as should women who have had past problems with birth control pills. The American Heart Association says ERT should be used cautiously in women with high triglycerides.

However, NYU's Dr. Nachtigall says *some* of these women may be permitted to use the transdermal patch or estrogen cream on the advice of their physician.

The American Heart Association's new Scientific Statement on Cardiovascular Disease in Women concludes that if a woman has a lower-than-average risk of heart disease, the decision whether to use HRT should be based on issues such as menopausal symptoms and osteoporosis. Many experts argue that if you have *no* adverse symptoms of menopause, such as hot flashes, if you're not at risk for osteoporosis and your cholesterol is low, you do not *need* to consider postmenopausal estrogen.

Some women sail through menopause with few symptoms and don't feel they need estrogen. Other women are not considered prime candidates for osteoporosis—those at high risk include fair-skinned women of northern European descent. For women who do not need or want estrogen, a physician may prescribe a diet low in fat and regular weight-bearing exercise (like walking) to keep lipid levels in check and to help preserve bone density.

BEWARE THE "MAGIC PILL" SYNDROME

It should be clear by now that, although hormone replacement has many benefits, HRT is not a magic pill that will totally eliminate your risk of heart disease.

Estrogen will not reduce the risks of smoking if you smoke; it will not lower your cholesterol or your weight if you habitually eat high-fat fast-foods, stresses Dr. Nachtigall.

If you stop taking hormones once you start, it's believed that the heart protection stops, too. Some women discontinue HRT because of side effects, such as menstrual-like bleeding, mood swings similar to premenstrual syndrome, weight gain and breast tenderness. Or they may skip a dose or a patch in an attempt to lessen symptoms. In that case, hormone therapy will probably not be as effective for them, and lifestyle changes, like exercise, may be a better alternative.

In general, most experts say the heart-saving benefits of hormone-replacement therapy far outweigh the risks, especially at the doses given to prevent osteoporosis or cardiovascular disease. But only you and your physician can determine if HRT is right for you.

11

Recognizing Signs
of Trouble

FOR MEN, a heart attack is often the first sign of heart disease. In women, the most common symptom is the chest pain or pressure known as *angina*. Women also suffer more "silent" heart attacks than men, leading to dangerous delays in diagnosing damage to the heart and increasing the risk of a second, more deadly, attack.

Being able to recognize what may be signs of heart disease or an imminent heart attack will help you to protect your heart from further damage and obtain the best medical care available, should you need it.

It should be stressed that the symptoms described in this chapter are offered as a guide to increase your awareness of potential problems, and are not a substitute for a professional medical diagnosis.

COMMON SYMPTOMS OF HEART DISEASE

According to Adina Kalet, M.D., M.P.H., a physician in the Division of Primary Care at NYU Medical Center, and director of Training Programs at NYU's Gouverneur Hospital Diagnostic Treatment Center, the symptoms which most often bring women into her office for an evaluation of possible heart disease are a feeling of pressure in the chest (angina), rapid heartbeats (palpitations) and shortness of breath during normal activities.

Older women, in particular, may suffer from shortness of breath, general tiredness or a near-fainting episode. Other symptoms may include dizziness, extreme fatigue and swelling of the ankles.

"Don't feel foolish or apologetic about seeing a doctor about any symptom, especially chest pressure or tightness, palpitations or shortness of breath," warns Dr. Kalet. "Don't wait to see a doctor if you experience sudden chest pain, especially during exercise. Even a momentary episode of weakness or trouble speaking can be a sign of trouble."

Statistics show that just as many women as men have heart attacks, but women may be less likely to report their symptoms to a physician— one reason why many heart attacks go unrecognized. Angina or other symptoms of coronary artery disease in women may also be dismissed by physicians because they sound "vague," or occur more often during emotional upsets than a man's. In addition, a 1994 survey found that many older people were unaware of the warning signs of heart failure, the leading cause of death and hospitalization among Americans age sixty-five and older. That's why it's important to know what symptoms may actually feel like, so that you can accurately describe them to a doctor.

Chest Pain/Angina: For more than 50 percent of women with coronary artery disease, *angina pectoris* (chest pressure or pain) is the first warning sign of heart trouble.

Angina occurs when the heart muscle is not getting adequate oxygen. Blood flow to the heart may be hampered by atherosclerotic plaques, a blood clot or a spasm in the coronary artery. When the heart demands more oxygen than it is getting, it stimulates pain fibers in the heart muscle to produce the discomfort of angina.

Angina usually occurs during moments of increased exertion or anxiety, when stress hormones constrict blood vessels, boost blood pressure and cause the heart to beat faster. Think of how your heart races and pressure seems to increase in your chest when you're late and running to catch a bus. Angina is also known to come on after a heavy meal, when extra blood and oxygen are being dispatched to the stomach and digestive tract so they can tackle the extra load. If a coronary artery blockage is severe enough, angina can also occur when a person is doing absolutely nothing.

The *difference* between angina and a heart attack is that during angina, there is still blood flowing to the heart; in a heart attack, blood flow is completely blocked. During angina, the heart muscles are painfully crying out for more oxygen, but unlike in a heart attack, areas of muscle do not die. Once normal blood flow resumes, heart cells resume their normal functions.

Anginal pain may last less than fifteen minutes; heart attack pain is more severe, lasting much longer (often with other symptoms described below), and does not go away with rest. However, angina may also be a sign that a heart attack is *imminent*.

For some women, angina symptoms may be predictable with certain activities. This is referred to as *stable angina*. If angina occurs with increasing frequency, or suddenly during rest, it's called *unstable angina*. Unstable angina is more common among women and is the most frequent cause of admissions to coronary care units.

In other cases, there may be no symptoms of inadequate blood flow to the heart, or *ischemia*. A 1994 study found silent ischemia to be a *better* predictor for fatal cardiovascular disease in older women than older men. People with diabetes may also be more prone to silent ischemia, possibly because of peripheral nerve damage.

Another form of angina, *Prinzmetal's* or *variant angina*, stems from spasms in coronary arteries, temporarily slowing blood flow. If the spasms are severe enough (or if you already have blockages in these arteries) a heart attack could occur. Only 1 to 2 percent of people with angina have this specific form of chest pain. It's much more common among women and hits at an earlier age than angina caused by coronary blockages. It is not triggered by exercise and comes on at rest, even during sleep. A major risk factor is cigarette smoking.

What Angina May Feel Like: Since angina symptoms may come and go, it's important to keep track of when they occur and what the symptoms feel like.

Some women describe angina as a feeling of tightness or pressure in the center of the chest, almost as if the heart were being squeezed by a giant fist. Many patients will actually make a fist and press it over the left side of their chest when describing their symptoms, a gesture physicians call the "Anginal Salute." This more subtle feeling of tightness or pressure may be more common than actual chest pain.

Anginal pain can radiate to the shoulders and down the inside of the arms (especially the left arm), or may spread to the jaw and feel like the sharp twinge of a toothache. The pain begins gradually and subsides with rest. The discomfort of angina may not always be painful, however. If the pain is especially sharp, is relieved by movement or is made worse by touching the chest, it may not be due to ischemia.

Angina can also feel like a burning sensation in the chest, but that symptom may be due to heartburn (where stomach acid leaks into the esophagus) or other digestive problems. If the pain worsens when you lie down (causing more stomach acid to seep into the esophagus), it's most likely heartburn. Only your doctor can determine if your pain stems from ischemia, heartburn, gallbladder disease or even an ulcer. Variant angina is not related to exercise and may wake you from a sound sleep.

Chest pain may also be caused by extreme anxiety, inflammation of the sac surrounding the heart or pericardium, pulmonary embolisms and lung disorders.

New federal guidelines for treating unstable angina, issued in 1994 by the National Heart, Lung and Blood Institute and the Agency for Health Care Policy Research, advise that anyone suffering unexpected, severe chest pains see a doctor at once. The guidelines also recommend calling an ambulance, then your doctor, if chest pain lasts more than twenty minutes and is accompanied by weakness, nausea and fainting and is not helped by three nitroglycerin tablets.

MARGERY'S STORY

"I woke up one morning with pain in my left side, in the chest. It felt like somebody was pulling all the muscles out.

"They took a cardiogram, but it was normal. They took a chest X-ray and it was normal. So they told me I probably had pleurisy and sent me home with anti-inflammatory drugs.

"But I still got the pain about three or four times a week, mostly at night. It would wake me up when I was sleeping. Sometimes during the day, it would just hit—it would intensify to the point where you couldn't stand it. Then it would subside. I kept asking for more anti-inflammatory drugs, more pain killers.

"The doctor kept repeating cardiograms. He was suspicious; he was the one who said, 'There's something wrong with her heart.' But nothing showed up on the EKG.

"After about two and a half or three months of walking around with this pain, it started to change. I felt the pain all down my left arm and in the right jaw, with the pain in the left chest. On Christmas Eve, I was up all night long in pain. When I finally called the doctor, he said, 'Get yourself to the hospital.' They found two coronary artery blockages."

Shortness of Breath/Dyspnea: Shortness of breath (medically referred to as *dyspnea*) can be an early warning sign of heart disease, particularly congestive heart failure (see page 196).

In congestive heart failure, the heart muscle has trouble pumping because it has been weakened by lack of oxygen due to clogged arteries, chronic high blood pressure, serious cardiac arrhythmias or heart valve disease. When too little blood is pumped from the heart, pressure builds in the lungs.

Shortness of breath, especially while lying down, is a major symptom of congestive heart failure on the left side of the heart. Oxygenated blood from the lungs travels from the lungs into the left atrium and then to the left ventricle, which pumps it out to the rest of the body. When this side of the heart isn't pumping properly, pressure builds up in the lungs, causing a backup of blood and fluid in the lungs, making a person feel short of breath. Pressure may also cause fluid to leak into the air sacs of the lungs, making breathing even more difficult.

If a valve between the heart's pumping chambers becomes diseased or narrowed, it can slow blood flow and trigger the same buildup of pressure.

What Dyspnea May Feel Like: Every woman has experienced temporary shortness of breath after hiking up a long flight of stairs with an armful of packages, especially women who are sedentary. However, when shortness of breath occurs during more moderate activity or at rest, it may be a sign of heart disease.

Shortness of breath may come gradually over time. Chronic shortness of breath is associated with congestive heart failure, especially when accompanied by extreme and sudden fatigue.

Chronic shortness of breath, with or without physical activity, is also a sign of heart valve disorders or lung disease. In lung disease, shortness of breath may be experienced as a difficulty getting air in and out of the lungs, with a tendency to take slower and deeper breaths. In cardiac dyspnea, a person tends to take rapid, shallow breaths.

Fainting/Syncope: It may have been expected for nineteenth-century ladies to fall into a swoon at the slightest upset, but these days, a fainting spell is taken quite seriously.

Fainting occurs when the brain is deprived of oxygen for more than ten seconds. When fainting is related to heart problems, it's called *cardiac syncope.* Cardiac syncope can often be triggered by heartbeat irregularities, which may hamper blood flow to the brain. Light-headedness can also accompany cardiac arrhythmias.

Fainting can also be a symptom of something called *Stokes-Adams Syndrome*, an interruption of electrical impulses in the heart, or *heart block*, resulting in inadequate blood supply to the brain.

An extremely slow heartbeat (fewer than thirty-five to forty-five beats per minute) can result in lowered blood pressure, and the brain will not get enough oxygen. People taking blood pressure medication may have a fainting spell if their pressure falls too low. Pregnant women can also experience fainting spells due to sudden drops in blood pressure.

A narrowing or obstruction in the arteries in the back of the neck, or *vertebral-basilar arteries*, which supply blood to the brain may cause fainting. In unusual cases, fainting can occur during a *transient ischemic attack* or *TIA*, which is actually a tiny stroke (see page 192).

What Cardiac Syncope May Feel Like: Light-headedness or dizziness may be the initial symptom. A person may not actually faint, but feel like the floor is slipping away from him, then recover before blacking out. If syncope results from a rapid heartbeat, chest pain and shortness of breath may also occur.

Feeling faint accompanied by dizziness, temporary weakness in the face or limbs on one side of the body, inability to speak, and unsteadiness in walking—these are usually signs that a TIA or a stroke has occurred.

NYU's Dr. Kalet notes that there are some people who faint easily at the sight of blood or with severe pain. This type of fainting spell is called a *vasovagal attack*, because it's caused by overstimulation of the vagus nerve, which helps control circulation, among other things. A vasovagal attack can be exacerbated by low blood volume or dehydration and mineral loss after exercise (you need to replenish water, salt and minerals with drinks designed for that purpose). In a vasovagal attack, fainting may be accompanied by heavy sweating or paleness of the skin, nausea, vomiting and slow heart rate.

Water Retention/Edema: Many women experience water retention, or *edema*, during the second half of their menstrual cycle. Edema can also occur late in pregnancy. These conditions are both temporary, related to a woman's hormones, not her heart.

However, chronic or sudden water retention with swelling in the ankles, legs, chest and abdomen can be a symptom of right-sided heart failure. When the right atrium and right ventricle aren't pumping efficiently, fluid and pressure build in the veins emptying into the right side of the heart. This forces excess fluid out of blood vessels into body tissues in the legs and abdomen.

What Heart-Related Edema May Feel Like: Ankle swelling that occurs regularly in the evening, making the skin around the ankles and feet feel tight, is a symptom of a more serious type of edema than is associated with premenstrual syndrome. If your ankles feel or look swollen, press your fingers into the skin just above the ankle bone. If an indentation remains for a moment after you remove your fingers, it's a sign of edema.

Uncomfortable and noticeable swelling or puffiness in the chest or abdominal wall, or swelling in the legs can be a sign of congestive heart failure and should be evaluated by a physician. Fluid in the abdomen may not be evenly distributed, and your flanks may feel swollen or sore from the added weight.

Palpitation: The heart beats an average of seventy-two times a minute, and most of the time, we go about our daily business completely unaware of it. Occasionally, however, the heart may start to beat hard and fast or seem to skip a beat for no apparent reason. It's a scary feeling and one of the most common reasons why women seek evaluation for heart disease.

Infrequent palpitations are usually nothing to worry about. We may become overly aware of the beating of our heart during times of heightened anxiety or stress; a pounding heartbeat may accompany a panic attack. Palpitations often occur at rest.

Sporadic palpitations can be thought of as tiny glitches in the heart's electrical system, explains Larry A. Chinitz, M.D., director of Cardiac Electrophysiology at NYU. Occasionally, an extra beat will set off a second heavy heartbeat in rapid succession. This is often called a *premature atrial contraction* and it can set off a series of palpitations.

According to Dr. Chinitz, these palpitations occur in healthy people and most often have no significant or long-term consequences. Occasional rapid heartbeats or extra beats can be triggered by vigorous exercise, drinking coffee or alcohol, smoking or even taking some prescription drugs.

Irregular or rapid beats that originate in the atrium and occur without physical exertion are called *supraventricular tachycardia* and are more common among women (see page 185). Most of the time, they are not related to heart disease, but should be checked out by a physician.

Palpitations may also be a symptom of mitral valve prolapse (see page 197), which affects twice as many women as men.

What Palpitations May Feel Like: Palpitations may range from a faint fluttering in the chest to a racing, pounding heartbeat that lasts a few seconds. It can be a single thump or a series of heavy beats, felt anywhere from the abdomen to the head.

Palpitations are often felt most keenly at night, while a woman is lying in bed in a quiet room. If the heart starts beating very rapidly for more than just a few minutes without heavy exertion, a person should seek medical evaluation. Avoiding emotional stress and anxiety, and stimulants such as caffeine may help some people control palpitations.

If palpitations become more frequent or severe or are accompanied by other symptoms, such as light-headedness, shortness of breath or fainting, it could be a sign of a more serious form of heart rhythm disturbance or arrhythmia. If you suffer from severe or frequent palpitations, consult a doctor.

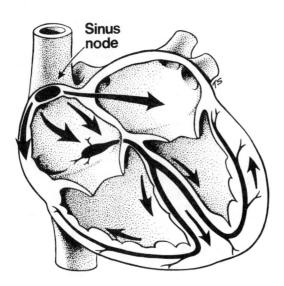

Source: The National Institutes of Health.

Cardiac Arrhythmias: While an occasional skipped beat can occur in a healthy heart, a damaged heart can produce more serious heart rhythm disturbances called *cardiac arrhythmias* (palpitation is a minor form of arrhythmia).

Arrhythmias are disruptions of the normal electrical sequence that regulates contraction of the heart muscle. In a healthy heart, the signal generated by the *sinoatrial* (SA) *node* (at the top of the right atrium) is sent through the atria to the *atrioventricular* (AV) *node*, located in the wall between the right and left ventricles. The AV node connects with special conducting fibers, which transmit the impulse to the right and then to the left pumping chambers, forcing blood down from the atria to the ventricles, then upward out to the body.

Other heart tissues are also capable of initiating a beat. When damage (such as a scar from a previous heart attack) blocks the normal conduction pathway, another part of the heart may be forced to take over as pacemaker. Abuse of drugs, especially alcohol and cocaine, can also interfere with heart rhythm. If the resulting heartbeat hampers blood flow, the outcome can be dangerous.

Arrhythmias can take the form of an abnormally slow heart rate known as *bradycardia*, fewer than sixty beats per minute, or a rapid heartbeat, *tachycardia*, of more than one hundred beats per minute. An abnormally slow heartbeat may mean that the heart is not able to pump blood to the body. An abnormally fast beat can reduce the heart's pumping capability by preventing the ventricles from filling properly, explains Dr. Chinitz.

The rapid heartbeats that originate in the upper chambers, supraventricular tachycardias, usually are not a symptom of heart disease, though sometimes they may need treatment. Rapid, irregular heartbeats that originate in the *lower* pumping chambers are called *ventricular tachycardia*, and these *are* most often associated with structural damage or heart disease.

Sometimes the heart's electrical system goes so haywire that several areas of heart tissue beat simultaneously. This is called *fibrillation*. When it occurs in the ventricles, it can be deadly. In *ventricular fibrillation*, cells in the lower chambers of the heart beat so chaotically, they cannot contract to pump blood out. Blood collects in the heart and unless immediate steps are taken to shock the heart back into its normal rhythm, a person may collapse and die. Ventricular fibrillation can occur with a heart attack.

If the upper chambers of the heart, or atria, start to fibrillate, blood flow through the heart can slow, and clots may form in stagnating blood. These can lodge in arteries that feed the brain. Atrial fibrillation causes 15 percent of all strokes (see page 193).

Atrial fibrillation appears to be a fairly common problem, affecting an estimated 3 percent of all Americans over sixty. It can be caused by congenital abnormalities, rheumatic heart disease, high blood pressure, or an overactive thyroid gland, but often there may be no discernible cause.

Some very active celebrants of Independence Day or New Year's Eve have been known to develop *holiday heart syndrome*—temporary atrial fibrillation brought on by excessive alcohol and lack of sleep.

In people with so-called *sick-sinus syndrome*, the heart's pacemaker slows due to disease, scarring of the heart, congenital heart defects or aging. This causes an abnormally slow pulse rate, sometimes alternating with a rapid rate, which diminishes output of blood.

Occasionally, people are born with extra electrical pathways in the heart, which eventually cause rapid heartbeats. One such condition, called *Wolff-Parkinson-White Syndrome*, can be controlled and, in some cases, cured with medical treatment.

What Cardiac Arrhythmias May Feel Like: Patients who have potentially serious cardiac arrhythmias will often have other symptoms such as light-headedness, dizziness or even loss of consciousness. They may develop shortness of breath or even chest pains, signs indicating the arrhythmias are occurring in the setting of some other structural heart abnormality. In some women, atrial fibrillation may feel like palpitations accompanied by light-headedness.

People with sick-sinus syndrome may experience fatigue, shortness of breath and even fainting spells due to lack of oxygen. Exercise may bring on these symptoms because the heart rate is not keeping pace with the body's activity.

Cardiac arrhythmias can be controlled with a variety of treatments, including pacemakers, which we'll discuss in Chapter 13.

PANIC ATTACK OR HEART ATTACK?

People who suffer from panic attacks often have symptoms mimicking heart attacks, fear they're having a heart attack, and often consult a doctor about chest pain. As many as one third to one half of patients who undergo tests for heart problems are found to have panic disorder.

Some three million Americans may suffer panic attacks at some point in their lives; panic disorder is twice as common among women as among men, and may also be associated with mitral valve prolapse (see page 197).

People suffering from panic disorder have unpredictable episodes of intense fear often accompanied by a pounding heart, chest pain, and shortness of breath, lasting from five to fifteen minutes. The diagnostic manual of the American Psychiatric Association classifies any person who suffers four or more such attacks in a given month as having panic disorder.

PHYSICAL SYMPTOMS OF PANIC ATTACKS

- Chest pain or discomfort
- Palpitations or rapid heartbeat
- Shortness of breath, feeling smothered or choked
- Dizziness, faintness, light-headedness
- Sweating, nausea or abdominal distress
- Trembling, numbness or tingling (especially in the hands)
- Hot flashes or chills

MENTAL SYMPTOMS OF PANIC ATTACKS

- Unprovoked terror; a sense that something horrible is about to happen and you are powerless to prevent it.
- Fear of having a heart attack or dying.
- Fear of going crazy or losing control.
- Perceptual distortions, dreamlike sensations, a sense of unreality, or feeling detached from your own experience.

SYMPTOMS OF HEART ATTACK/
MYCARDIAL INFARCTION

A quarter of a million American women die every year of heart attacks. Since most heart-attack deaths occur within the first hour or so of the attack—even before a woman reaches the hospital—recognizing the warning signs can make the difference between life and death.

It's estimated that up to 40 percent of women who've had heart attacks, or *myocardial infarctions,* had no symptoms, compared to less than 30 percent of men. Women most prone to "silent" heart attacks include those with diabetes and smokers. Some experts believe that peripheral nerve damage resulting from diabetes may suppress heart-attack symptoms; recent research suggests that nicotine may reduce sensitivity to pain.

In any case, up to 37 percent of heart attacks (even those with symptoms) may go unidentified in women.

Most heart attacks occur because an artery supplying the heart becomes completely blocked, usually by a blood clot (called a *coronary thrombosis*) that forms in an area narrowed by atherosclerotic plaque.

In other cases, a narrowed coronary artery may spasm, blocking blood flow to the heart, an occurrence more common in women than in men. Spasms can occur in diseased arteries, but they can also occur in healthy people. They can occur as a result of cocaine use and are also associated with smoking in women (snorting cocaine and smoking is an especially hazardous combination). Disease and certain congenital heart problems (such as aortic stenosis, or narrowing of the aorta) may also cause heart attacks.

Whatever the cause, when blood supply to the heart is cut off, heart muscle tissue is deprived of oxygen and irreparable cell damage can occur if blood flow is not restored. In some cases, drugs that dissolve blood clots given as soon as possible after a heart attack can minimize cell damage. Treatments that can prevent heart attacks (or head off a second attack) include angioplasty and coronary bypass surgery (see Chapter 13).

HELEN'S STORY

"I had absolutely no idea I was having a heart attack—I thought it was an upset stomach.

"My husband has had angina for twenty years, and he had just had a mild heart attack. We had taken him to the hospital and they were recommending a bypass. While my son and I were wrestling with that, I started to feel nauseous. I was throwing up. I thought it was from the worry about my husband.

"But it was so bad, I went right over to the doctor. He told me to drink ginger ale for the rest of the day. But he was concerned enough to take a lot of blood tests.

"We had theater tickets before all this happened, and my husband said I should go. So that night, I went with my son. The next day, we did all the errands. After supper, I started throwing up violently again, and I had very severe pains across my back. I often have severe arthritic pain, so I thought that's what it was. I'd had an ulcer last year and I thought maybe that was it. I took the heating pad and went to lie down. And I felt better.

"The next day, the doctor called and said the blood tests showed some abnormalities—very high cholesterol for one thing—and he said I should come right into the hospital. . . . On the way to the hospital [the vomiting] was so bad, I had to take a plastic bag in the car.

"In the emergency room, they told me I'd had a small heart attack, but fortunately, there had been only slight damage to the heart. I was shocked . . . I'd had no chest pains, no warning.

"But the doctor said that sometimes a heart attack comes and brings on the vomiting, or the vomiting is a precursor of it; they don't really know why. Another doctor pointed out that a buildup of coronary artery disease occurs over ten, twenty, thirty, even forty years. People don't realize it, but after menopause, women don't have the protection of estrogen. The buildup in the arteries can happen very fast. That's apparently what happened to me.

"My husband started having angina in his forties, and I had a heart attack at sixty-eight; I caught up with him. We ended up having bypass operations within two days of each other."

What a Heart Attack May Feel Like: The pain of a heart attack results from cramping of the heart muscle due to lack of oxygen. Most people mistakenly believe that a heart attack always feels like a sharp, stabbing pain in the left side of the chest. However, pressure in the chest may be the most common symptom. It is felt in the center of the chest, just behind the breastbone, and it can radiate to either shoulder, to the back, to the arms and often (but not always) to the left side.

Pain can also radiate to the jaw or the ears. Unlike angina, this pain will not subside when you stop whatever you're doing and rest. A woman having a heart attack will also feel pale, weak and short of breath, breaking into a cold sweat. She may feel dizzy, light-headed, feel palpitations or start to cough.

A person with previously diagnosed angina may find that a nitroglycerine tablet placed under the tongue brings only temporary relief from the pain. Frequent and severe angina attacks, especially at night or while resting, may be a sign of imminent heart attack. If you have been previously diagnosed with angina, take nitroglycerine as directed by your doctor. If the pain does not subside, call 911.

If you're a woman in middle age or just approaching it, don't think you can't be having a heart attack (especially if you have a family history of heart disease). Don't dismiss your discomfort as a sign of "aging," and don't "wait and see if it gets better." Studies show that women generally let as much as four hours lapse between the onset of their symptoms and calling for help, compared to an hour in men.

HEART ATTACK: SIGNALS AND ACTION

KNOW THE WARNING SIGNS OF A HEART ATTACK

- Uncomfortable pressure, fullness, squeezing or pain in the center of the chest lasting more than a few minutes, or goes away and comes back.
- Chest pain that spreads to the shoulders, neck or arms.
- Chest discomfort with light-headedness, fainting, weakness, sweating, nausea or shortness of breath.

Not all of these symptoms occur with every heart attack. But if some start to occur, don't wait. Get help immediately. Do not minimize or dismiss your symptoms. Delay can be deadly!

KNOW WHAT TO DO IN AN EMERGENCY

- Find out which area hospitals have twenty-four-hour emergency cardiac care.
- Know (in advance) which hospital or medical facility is nearest to your home and office, and tell your family and friends to call this facility in an emergency.
- Keep a list of emergency-rescue service numbers next to the telephone and in your pocket, wallet or purse.
- If you have chest discomfort that lasts ten minutes or more, call your local emergency-rescue service immediately.
- If you can get to the hospital faster by car, by going yourself and not waiting for an ambulance, have someone drive you. *Do not* attempt to drive yourself to the hospital.

BE A HEART SAVER

- If you're with someone who is experiencing signs of a heart attack—and the symptoms last more than a few minutes—act immediately.
- Expect a denial. It's normal for someone with chest discomfort to deny the possibility of something as serious as a heart attack. Don't take *no* for an answer. Insist on taking prompt action.

continued

- Call 911 (or your local emergency service) or get the person to the nearest hospital emergency room that offers twenty-four-hour cardiac care.
- Give CPR (mouth-to-mouth breathing and chest compression) —if it's necessary and you're properly trained.

If heart disease runs in your family, or if you or a family member have heart disease, it's a good idea to get CPR training. Classes are usually available through your local Red Cross or Y, or call the American Heart Association for information on CPR training in your area.

STROKES/TRANSIENT ISCHEMIC ATTACKS

Stroke is actually a form of cardiovascular disease that affects the blood vessels connecting the heart to the brain. Strokes, or *cerebrovascular disease*, can be caused by blood clots or burst blood vessels, both of which disrupt blood supply to the brain or parts of the brain. More than 60 percent of deaths from strokes are among women.

In some people, strokes occur because the blood platelets become "sticky." This can occur when there's too much of a substance called *fibrinogen* (which is naturally higher in women) that causes platelets to form clots.

When brain cells are deprived of oxygen, they die within minutes, and the parts of the body controlled by these cells become impaired. The disability varies according to the size of the area affected, but the effects of stroke are often permanent, because brain cells do not regenerate.

A majority of strokes are caused by *cerebral thrombosis*, a blood clot in an artery supplying part of the brain. Blood clots tend to form in arteries already clogged and damaged by atherosclerosis. The carotid arteries, the two main blood lines to the brain, are often affected. However, studies show women and blacks tend to have more blockages in the arteries in the head, the *intercranial arteries*, than men.

Cerebral thrombosis may often be preceded by a transient ischemic attack, or TIA, actually a tiny stroke, which temporarily clogs an artery and lasts less than five minutes. Because the blockage is so brief, people usually return to normal. However, a TIA is often an important warning sign: Some 36 percent of people who have had one or more TIAs go on to suffer a stroke.

From 5 to 14 percent of strokes are caused by a *cerebral embolism*, a blood clot formed in another part of the body (usually in the heart or from plaques in the aorta and its branches) which travels in the bloodstream until it lodges in an artery leading to or in the brain itself. These emboli are often formed during atrial fibrillation, in which the upper chambers of the heart quiver instead of pump effectively, so blood isn't pushed completely out of the atria. When blood stagnates, it tends to form clots.

Two kinds of brain hemorrhage also cause strokes. A *subarachnoid hemorrhage* occurs when a blood vessel on the surface of the brain ruptures and bleeds into the space between the skull and the brain. This type of hemorrhage does not cause bleeding inside the brain itself, but the bleeding and resulting clot can cause pressure on the brain. In a *cerebral hemorrhage*, a defective artery bursts inside the brain itself, flooding surrounding tissue with blood. In some cases, a blood clot can be removed surgically.

Brain hemorrhages can be caused by a burst aneurysm, a pouch that forms at a weak spot in an artery wall, often due to chronic high blood pressure. Head injuries also cause brain hemorrhage.

TIAs and ischemic strokes may be treated with use of anticoagulants, daily doses of aspirin or surgery to open blocked carotid arteries (see page 232).

What TIAs and Strokes May Feel Like: If you are having a TIA, you may experience a sudden weakness in one side of the body, in an arm or leg, or in the face. You may have trouble understanding what someone is saying and may be unable to speak yourself. Vision may be blurred or dimmed or you may not be able to see out of one eye. You may feel dizzy, unsteady on your feet, have difficulty walking or you may even fall down. You may have a sudden and severe headache.

Symptoms of a TIA can last less than five minutes or up to twenty-four hours, and then fade. But since TIAs are a key warning sign of an impending stroke, you need to see a doctor *as soon as possible.*

In a person having a stroke, these symptoms last much longer, and the person may be incapacitated or lose consciousness. Strokes require swift emergency medical care.

A sudden, excruciating headache is probably the most common symptom of a cerebral or subarachnoid hemorrhage, along with a feeling of faintness or loss of consciousness. There may also be nausea, vomiting, dizziness, intellectual impairment or seizures.

If you're experiencing one or more of these symptoms (or you're with someone else who is), get immediate medical attention. Call an ambulance or have someone call one for you. Do *not* wait. Only a physician can determine if you have had a TIA, stroke or have some other medical condition with similar symptoms.

It should be noted that these ministrokes may also be the cause of many cases of "senile dementia" in the elderly, which might be mistaken for Alzheimer's disease. A recent study in the *New England Journal of Medicine* reported that out of nearly five hundred people of age eighty-five screened for dementia, almost *half* had had multiple TIAs. The important message here is that many cases of vascular dementia could be *prevented* by prompt treatment of TIAs, atrial fibrillation, and stroke-reduction measures such as smoking cessation and controlling high blood pressure.

RUTH'S STORY

"My grandmother was in her eighties and had been treated for high blood pressure for many years when she started having TIAs. I was with her during one episode; I remember it vividly. It was after lunch, and we were sitting there having tea and her special cookies.

"I remember she was handing me the cookie jar, and whatever she was saying started to sound garbled. Her arm just flopped down with the cookie jar and I saw the side of her face go slack. I knew immediately she was having a stroke. I ran to the phone to call 911. She blacked out and fell off her chair while I was calling the ambulance.

"I helped her up and told her an ambulance was on the way. She appeared to recover her senses and started arguing with me that this was nothing; it had happened before. 'Call them back and tell them not to come. It's just old age,' she insisted. But the EMS crew was already at the door.

"She later admitted to the doctors that she had had maybe three or four similar incidents over a period of a year or so; they hadn't lasted long, and she'd just gone about her business afterward. She had become increasingly forgetful during that time. She lived alone and was fiercely independent. During one TIA, she fell and had badly cut her head, but told no one.

"They put her on blood thinners and reassured us there was no lasting brain damage; but the next time she might not be so lucky. There might be a possible blockage in one of the neck arteries, and they advised her to go for further tests, but she never did. She had several more TIAs and died from an apparent stroke a couple of years later at age eighty-nine. I miss her a lot.

"What I'd like to tell women like my grandmother is: Never, never dismiss an episode like that as 'just aging.' Don't be afraid to get help."

CONGESTIVE HEART FAILURE

As many as three million Americans suffer from heart failure—but it's not always fatal. "The term *heart failure* does not mean the heart has stopped beating . . . but rather, that it can't pump enough blood to meet the demands of the body," says Sydney J. Mehl, M.D., clinical associate professor of medicine at NYU. Because heart failure often results in a buildup of fluid in the lungs, it's also referred to as congestive heart failure.

Since the weakened heart also can't deliver enough blood to the kidneys, the kidneys don't excrete excess salt and water. These accumulate in tissues, causing swelling.

The most common cause of congestive heart failure is a heart attack or ischemia. Atherosclerosis can produce heart failure by depriving the heart of oxygen it needs.

A leaky valve or too-tight heart valve can also interfere with the heart's ability to pump effectively, and an overactive thyroid can contribute to heart failure. Too much thyroid hormone or too little can have effects on cardiac function, explains Dr. Mehl.

In general, heart failure is caused by ineffective muscle contraction, and drugs can be given to strengthen the pumping action of the heart. The most severe cases of heart failure are caused by scarring of the heart after heart attacks, or by diseases of the heart muscle. The ultimate treatment in such cases is a heart transplant.

What Heart Failure May Feel Like: A woman with heart failure may find herself fatigued by normal activity, feeling worse as the day wears on and perhaps totally exhausted by evening. Her legs may feel weak or heavy. The exhaustion may be so complete, she may feel as if she can't even think straight.

Because of fluid accumulating in lungs and tissues, she may also be short of breath, have uncomfortably swollen legs or may feel very bloated. She may have difficulty breathing at night or upon awakening. If there is congestion in the lungs, she may cough up sputum tinged with blood. In some cases, the skin will become cyanotic, develop a bluish cast. These symptoms can come on fairly suddenly and should prompt an immediate visit to a physician.

LAURA'S STORY

"It was around the time I was planning my wedding when I started to feel some strange and unusual symptoms: my heart would suddenly race and pound in my chest. I'd have chest pain. I was short of breath and would become extremely fatigued. I would have these attacks of sheer panic; I felt like I was going to die or collapse and I had to escape from wherever I was.

"The doctors listened to my heart, but said there was nothing wrong. They felt my problem might be neurological, but magnetic resonance imaging turned up nothing wrong there. But it kept on getting worse. I had one panic attack that was so bad, I ended up in the emergency room; I really believed I was going to die. I say 'panic attacks' now, because I now know what they were. Back then, I had no idea what was happening to me.

"I must have seen six doctors over a few months. Some suggested it was just stress and told me not to drink coffee. One prescribed ulcer medication. Another doctor strongly implied . . . that I was imagining it, which made me furious! But since no one could find anything wrong, I almost started to believe him.

"Finally, my husband suggested I see his physician, who happened to be a woman. She listened, really listened to what had been happening to me. She didn't hear a heart murmur, but she suspected mitral valve prolapse. She ordered an echocardiogram, and that confirmed it. She also put me on a holter monitor for twenty-four hours to check how my heart was functioning. She put me on medication to control my rapid heartbeats, and I've been on it now for five years.

"Just knowing what it was, that I didn't have some fatal heart condition or was going crazy, was such a tremendous relief! I've learned that mitral valve prolapse is a condition that mostly affects women. I think the doctors should have been more aware that even a young woman could have a heart problem. They made me feel as if I really did have a psychological, not a physical, problem."

MITRAL VALVE PROLAPSE

It's not known why, but more women than men are born with some sort of congenital heart defect. Some defects obstruct the flow of blood to the heart or nearby blood vessels, others cause abnormal blood flow through the heart.

As many as 6 percent of all women may have *mitral valve prolapse*, or MVP. The rate of occurrence is almost three times higher among women between the ages of twenty and forty, and MVP tends to run in families.

The mitral valve is made of two flaps or "leaflets" that guard the opening between the left atrium and the left ventricle, the upper and lower chambers on the left side of the heart. In a normal heart, when blood leaves the left atrium it flows through the mitral valve into the left ventricle. When the left ventricle contracts, the mitral valve snaps shut to prevent blood from flowing back into the atrium.

In people with mitral valve prolapse, the valve leaflets become enlarged or may become misshapen with extra tissue. Instead of closing tightly, they flop backward and allow blood to seep back into the atrium when the left ventricle contracts. This seepage produces the murmur or clicking sound characteristic of MVP that can be heard with a stethoscope. The click alone can be a sign of MVP, even if there's no leakage.

The disorder is usually not serious, although in rare cases, it can cause more severe leakage of the valve and subsequent enlargement of the heart muscle. In such cases, the valve may need to be replaced or repaired surgically.

Mitral valve prolapse may make a woman more susceptible to *bacterial endocarditis*, an infection of the heart valves, since damaged valves are more prone to infections. The bacteria may get into the bloodstream during medical or dental procedures that cause bleeding as well as during childbirth (see page 201). If a woman is known to have MVP, antibiotics are given before surgery and dental procedures. The disorder is often first diagnosed when a woman becomes pregnant.

The disorder is usually diagnosed with an echocardiogram, ultrasound pictures of the heart. While most women require no treatment for MVP, low doses of antiarrhythmic drugs may be used to control frequent palpitations.

Infrequently, MVP may lead to serious arrhythmias, or small blood clots may form on the defective valves and cause TIAs.

What Mitral Valve Prolapse May Feel Like: Many women with MVP report mild palpitations or skipped heartbeats, but other women have vague symptoms or none at all. In some cases, women may have minor chest pain, thought to be due to a stretching of the tissue connecting the mitral leaflets to small muscles on the valve, called papillary muscles, depriving them of oxygen.

Occasionally MVP can cause some light-headedness, dizziness, shortness of breath, numbness or even fainting. These kinds of symptoms could be associated with TIAs and should be reported to a physician immediately.

MVP has also been associated with anxiety attacks or panic (see page 187), although just why is not clear, so some women may need to be treated with antianxiety medication.

PREGNANCY AND HEART DISEASE

More and more women are delaying childbearing until their forties, so heart disease may complicate a pregnancy. Cardiovascular disease can make pregnancy difficult and risky without careful medical supervision.

Women diagnosed with hypertension before they became pregnant are considered high-risk pregnancies, but may experience relatively few problems if their pressure is kept under control. Most antihypertensive medications are considered relatively safe during pregnancy, with the exception of ACE inhibitors. A woman with extremely high blood pressure may need to be hospitalized for a brief period during pregnancy.

Peripartum Cardiomyopathy: Women with hypertension may be at increased risk for peripartum cardiomyopathy, a relatively rare inflammation of the heart muscle that can occur during the last month of pregnancy or within a few months of delivery. Recent research suggests that the inflammation may be the result of an autoimmune response, where the immune system produces antibodies to attack cells or chemicals it perceives as foreign invaders.

In this case, the trigger may be contractile proteins produced by muscle cells in the uterus preparation for labor and delivery. These proteins are very similar to contractile proteins in heart cells. So when this autoimmune response is triggered, the heart muscle is attacked in addition to the proteins in the bloodstream. The left ventricle is especially affected. If the damage becomes severe enough, it can lead to heart failure. However, if the damage is slight, the ventricle may return to normal within six months of delivery.

Peripartum cardiomyopathy is treated with a combination of bed rest, salt restriction (to reduce edema), diet and occasionally immunosuppressant drugs, which hamper immune responses. Women who survive a bout with this disease are at a very high risk for a recurrence during subsequent pregnancies.

In addition to women with high blood pressure, pregnant women at increased risk for peripartum cardiomyopathy include women over age thirty-five, those carrying twins and women who have an extremely poor diet. African-American women are particularly at risk for this disorder.

What Peripartum Cardiomyopathy May Feel Like: Fatigue is a familiar sensation for many women both during pregnancy and shortly afterward. But becoming exhausted with the slightest exertion and feeling short of breath may be a warning sign of peripartum cardiomyopathy. The condition may also trigger rapid heartbeats. Some women will have severe swelling of the feet.

Pregnancy-Induced Hypertension/Preeclampsia: As mentioned in Chapter 3, one quarter of otherwise healthy expectant mothers may develop temporary *pregnancy-induced hypertension.* Only about 6 percent of these women develop the condition known as *preeclampsia.*

During pregnancy, a woman's blood volume increases by as much as 50 percent, to keep mother and baby supplied with oxygen and vital nutrients. In most healthy women, hormones are produced that help blood vessels expand and contract with increased blood flow. It's believed that in some women, an imbalance of these hormones leads to increased vasoconstriction and preeclampsia.

Left untreated, it can progress to *eclampsia,* a condition that can cause seizures, organ failure, coma and even the death of the mother. However, only about 5 percent of women with preeclampsia progress to this point. Eclampsia impairs blood flow to the fetus, which can cause many problems with growth and development. The baby may have to be delivered before term, risking still more complications.

In extreme cases, eclampsia may cause *abruptio placentae,* where blood vessels leading to the placenta weaken and cause it to tear away from the uterine wall. This can trigger hemorrhage in the mother and the premature birth of her baby.

What Preeclampsia May Feel Like: Warning signs of preeclampsia include fluid retention, swelling of the face, hands, feet or lower legs, and weight gain over two pounds during a single week. An expectant mother may also experience a headache that lingers for hours, as well as blurred vision or dizziness and occasionally pain in the upper abdomen.

Pregnant women are given regular blood pressure checks as well as urine tests for elevated amounts of a protein called albumin, a sign of preeclampsia.

Valvular Stenosis: If a woman has had rheumatic fever in the past, she may develop problems with heart valves scarred by the disease. These problems may manifest themselves for the first time during pregnancy, when maternal blood flow is increased.

Valvular stenosis is a thickening, narrowing or distortion of the heart valves due to the strep infection that causes rheumatic fever. The valves most commonly affected are the mitral valve (between the left atrium and the left ventricle) and the aortic valve (between the left ventricle and the aorta).

In *mitral stenosis*, a severely narrowed mitral valve may cause a backup of blood in the lungs, causing fluid buildup. In *aortic stenosis*, or constriction of the aortic valve, blood flow from the left ventricle into the aorta may be impaired, putting a strain on the heart.

What Valvular Stenosis May Feel Like: Symptoms of aortic stenosis include shortness of breath or difficulty breathing, dizziness, fainting or angina. In mitral stenosis, a woman may have shortness of breath accompanied by fatigue and coughing.

Bacterial Endocarditis: A woman who has heart-valve defects or rheumatic fever may also be at risk of developing *bacterial endocarditis.* This is an infection that may occur when bacteria enters a woman's body during bleeding episodes during delivery. To prevent this, cardiologists may prescribe antibiotics at the time of delivery for women with previously diagnosed valve abnormalities.

Women with other heart problems may also have to switch medication, since even drugs that are considered safe during pregnancy can still have side effects. Certain drugs, especially aspirin, ACE inhibitors (including enalapril and captopril), the cholesterol-lowering drug lovastatin are also not recommended for use during pregnancy. Most diuretics are allowed, if used before pregnancy. Clinical experience with some medications during pregnancy is limited, and a woman's physician must weigh the benefits against possible risks to the baby.

In some cases, a woman's doctor may strongly advise against pregnancy. A weakened heart may not be able to cope with the increased demands and the expanded blood volume of pregnancy; a woman's heart must work progressively harder to pump blood as the baby grows and needs more oxygen and nutrients. Heart rate and blood pressure also increase during labor and delivery. Use of epidural or spinal anesthesia can help stabilize heart output and blood pressure, or a cesarean delivery may be advised to lessen the strain on the heart. After delivery, when extra blood is no longer being sent to the fetus, a woman's blood volume surges temporarily, which could stress a weakened heart.

However, today many women with cardiovascular problems are able to have uneventful pregnancies and deliver healthy babies with careful monitoring by both an obstetrician and cardiologist.

12

Investigating Trouble

IF YOU ARE experiencing symptoms of heart disease, your doctor will probably order one or more diagnostic tests. This chapter will clarify current tests and treatments, so you can make informed decisions about which may be appropriate for you.

DIAGNOSING HEART DISEASE

In women, early physical symptoms of heart disease (such as chest pressure) are often too subtle for a physician to make a definitive diagnosis. A series of diagnostic tests can determine if there is a problem, how extensive it is and what needs to be done to correct it. These tests may include:

Electrocardiogram (EKG or ECG): An EKG is a quick, painless, non-invasive test that provides a record of the electric currents generated by the heart, while the patient is at rest. It's commonly used as a "baseline" against which to measure future EKGs or heart activity during exertion. A woman over age sixty-five with a family history of heart disease or other cardiac risk factors will often have an EKG as part of a routine medical exam.

WHAT YOUR EKG SHOWS

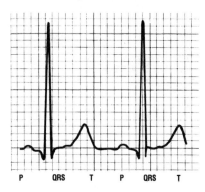

P   QRS   T   P   QRS   T

This EKG shows two complete normal heart cycles or sequence of contractions in a full, normal heartbeat. P shows the electrical signal that causes contraction of the heart. QRS shows the signal of the ventricles. T is the heart's return to its resting state. (Source: National Heart, Lung and Blood Institute)

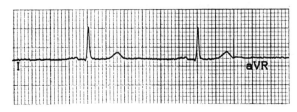

In this EKG, the heart cycle is slower, with too much time elapsing between contractions, possibly leading to inadequate heart function. The diagnosis is Sinus Bradycardia. (Source: Dr. Larry Chinitz, NYU Medical Center)

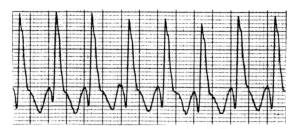

As this EKG illustrates, the heartbeat is rapid, with too little time between contractions. The diagnosis is Sinus Tachycardia. (Source: Dr. Larry Chinitz, NYU Medical Center)

To perform the test, ten electrodes are placed on areas of the chest, arms and legs after a special jellylike conductive material is applied. Electrical impulses from the heart chambers are picked up by the electrodes and sent through wires into the electrocardiograph machine, to be printed out on graph paper, which shows electrical patterns in the atria and ventricles. The resulting patterns on the graphs show whether the heart rhythm is regular. The test itself takes about thirty seconds.

Because an EKG is taken at rest, it won't detect problems in most people with symptoms of angina (unless the patient is having an attack of ischemia at the time). However, it can detect rhythm disturbances or damage from a previous, perhaps "silent," heart attack.

Holter Monitoring: When more information is needed about the heart's activity, a patient may be asked to wear a Holter monitor. This consists of a portable EKG and cassette recording device, worn for twenty-four hours. Electrodes attached to the chest feed information onto a special recorder, which is scanned through a computer, then printed out on graph paper just like a regular EKG. A woman is also asked to keep a log of her activities, which can be compared with the data to see whether certain activities trigger specific problems.

Holter monitoring can pick up episodes of silent ischemia and potentially dangerous arrhythmias that may not have shown up during a resting EKG. Your doctor may ask you to wear a Holter monitor if you're complaining of frequent or severe palpitations, chest pains, dizziness or fainting spells.

Exercise Stress Test: This is an EKG taken during exercise, which is then measured against a resting EKG.

First, the resting EKG and blood pressure are taken. The patient then exercises on a treadmill or exercise bicycle while hooked up to the electrocardiograph machine. The patient gradually increases the level of exercise to a target heart rate based on her physical condition and age (usually, to at least 85 percent of the maximum heart rate), until chest pains or other symptoms occur, or changes are seen in the EKG. Blood pressure is also monitored.

If the arteries are narrowed or in spasm and parts of the heart muscle do not get enough blood, it might show up on the graph as a depression of the S-T segment (as the ventricles finish pumping blood out to the body, and the heart "recharges" for another beat). According to Itzhak Kronzon, M.D., director of Noninvasive Cardiology at NYU, if changes in the EKG or symptoms like chest pain show up after just a few minutes or at a fairly low heart rate, this can mean that a patient has severe coronary artery disease (CAD).

However, this test cannot detect the earliest symptoms of CAD. Problems may not be seen unless one or more coronary arteries is at least 50 percent blocked. The test can also detect cardiac arrhythmias that occur during exertion or stress.

In general, about 65 percent of patients who have heart disease will be correctly diagnosed with a stress test. However, the false positive rate can be as high as 15 to 40 percent in women (especially before menopause). One reason suggested for this is that women may have different physiological responses to exercise than men.

The new American Heart Association Scientific Statement on Cardiovascular Disease in Women recommends that women with minimal or atypical angina who have a normal resting EKG be given an exercise stress test. If results are normal, no further testing may be needed. If results are abnormal, the AHA recommends ultrasound stress tests, or studies using radioactive materials to trace blood flow in the heart, should be done to be sure the test was not a false positive.

Echocardiogram: An echocardiogram uses ultrasound to take a two-dimensional, detailed picture of the structure of the heart as it beats. A special conduction gel is applied, and a transducer or wand is passed over various areas of the chest, emitting high-frequency sound waves that bounce off heart structures. The woman lies on her left side during the test, which takes about thirty minutes.

Echocardiography can pinpoint functional problems while the heart is actually beating, and can detect blood clots, valvular problems, heart enlargement and thickening of the heart muscle.

In some cases, *Doppler* ultrasound may be added. This measures changes in the sound waves produced by changes or abnormalities in blood flow through the heart's chambers. It also gauges heart valve pressure to check for narrowing or leakage.

The newest technique in cardiac ultrasound, now being used at NYU, is intravascular ultrasound, in which a miniature transducer is used to actually see inside coronary arteries and show the exact location and nature of fatty plaques. Another new procedure is called *transesophageal echocardiography*, in which the sonar wand is attached to a long, flexible tube and (under local anesthesia) inserted into the esophagus. It provides detailed pictures from the back of the heart and can often see valve problems more clearly and more accurately spot blood clots in areas where they're likely to be lurking.

Echo-Stress Test: This test combines ultrasound technology with an exercise stress test, and may be especially helpful for detecting heart problems in women.

Ultrasound pictures of the heart are first taken at rest, then entered into a computer. The woman will then be put on a treadmill (or an exercise bike) and asked to exercise to a predetermined heart rate (or until symptoms occur). Ultrasound pictures of the heart are then taken while the heart is still stressed. The computerized resting and stress images are then compared.

"During an echo-stress test, we can actually see the motion of the walls of the heart during exercise. In a healthy person, the heart not only beats faster during exercise, but the functioning of the heart's chambers improves," explains Dr. Kronzon. "If a segment of the heart is not receiving enough blood, its motion will be impaired. This shows up before there is chest pain and before an abnormal EKG."

Since women are more likely to have a false positive (or false negative) result from a conventional stress test, the echo-stress test can often provide a more definitive diagnosis. It can show obstruction to blood flow to the heart, if there is a weakness or scarring of the heart wall and whether normal amounts of blood are being pumped from the ventricles (called the *ejection fraction*). It can also reveal valve problems, including mitral valve prolapse, which are more common in women.

Thallium Stress Test: This exercise stress test introduces the element of blood-flow imaging. A small amount of a radioactive substance such as *thallium* is injected into the bloodstream. Once carried to the heart, it is absorbed by heart muscle. The dose of radiation is minuscule, and thallium is not considered harmful.

Radioactive thallium gives off *gamma rays*, and a *gamma camera* scans the heart's uptake of the radioisotope. The gamma rays "light up" in the resulting images of the heart muscle where thallium is taken up along with blood, explains Stephen A. Siegel, M.D., assistant director of NYU's Cardiac Stress Lab.

The procedure is almost the same as an exercise stress test, except that the patient is given an intravenous infusion of glucose (sugar and water) at the start of the exercise period. When the patient approaches the target rate (or when symptoms appear), the thallium is injected, and the patient exercises for another sixty seconds. She then lies down while the gamma camera takes pictures. After two to three hours of rest, another set of photos is taken of the heart. A third set of pictures, if needed, is taken twenty-four hours later. Together, these pictures will show if ischemia is present or whether there's been damage to the heart, and how extensive it may be. "Healthy heart muscle will literally be glowing all over. If a section of the heart isn't getting enough blood supply because of blockages in the artery, it will appear darker. After three hours, if the thallium isn't taken up evenly by the muscle, it means there has been some damage to the heart muscle," says Dr. Siegel. "If the pictures show inadequate thallium uptake both during exercise and while at rest, it's an indication there may be permanent damage."

If a woman is unable to exercise adequately (due to other illnesses like arthritis, medication or deconditioning), a *nonexercise* stress test can be performed. This test uses drugs to simulate the effects of exercise, increasing heart rate, and blood pressure, or to dilate blood vessels (healthy blood vessels will let more blood through; unhealthy vessels will not dilate).

Thallium stress tests are generally about 90 percent accurate in both sexes, and may be recommended when the results of a standard exercise stress test are inconclusive.

However, a woman's breast tissue may interfere with imaging, and the resulting shadows may appear similar to a blockage, notes Dr. Siegel. There is also a condition known as *microvascular angina* (sometimes called *Syndrome X*), which is more common among women. In cases of Syndrome X, no blockages can be detected in major coronary arteries; the problem may be with much smaller blood vessels. So a thallium stress test may come up positive, when the problem lies elsewhere.

MUGA Scans: Like the thallium stress test, this test traces small amounts of a radioisotope (in this case, *technetium pyrophosphate*) through the heart. But this test, called a *multigated acquisition scan,* or MUGA *scan,* provides a stop-action sequence of blood cells flowing through the chambers of the heart, and gives a very accurate measurement of how much blood is being ejected with each beat. Each stage in the beat sequence can be examined separately or in motion by computer.

MUGA scans are usually done when a physician suspects a problem with the heart's main pumping chamber, the left ventricle. These scans can see how much blood is being ejected from the left ventricle, or detect problems associated with problems of heart-muscle function, among them, congestive heart failure and congenital heart defects.

PET Scans: A more expensive but possibly more beneficial test for women may be *positron emission tomography*, or *PET* scans. Unlike thallium tests, PET scans are not affected by breast tissue. PET scans use tiny amounts of radioactive isotopes to image energy metabolism and blood perfusion in the heart. PET scans create sharp, three-dimensional pictures of the heart. Although it is still investigational, the technology may become more widely used in the future.

Cardiac Catheterization and Angiography: Cardiac catheterization involves inserting a thin plastic tube (a catheter) into a blood vessel, usually in the groin area or the arm, and gently passing it up into the heart. This is done under local anesthesia, generally in a hospital setting.

Several tests can be performed using catheterization. The most common is called *coronary angiography:* injecting a small amount of *radio-opaque dye* through the catheter and then taking "X-ray movies" as it flows through the coronary arteries into the heart, explains Dr. Siegel. Because dye blocks X rays, it appears opaque in the blood vessels, clearly showing any area that is narrowed or blocked. The X-ray pictures can also determine if smaller blood vessels, called collateral blood vessels, have formed to provide an alternate route to the heart. To observe the left side of the heart, the catheter is inserted through a leg artery; to observe the right side of the heart, a vein is used.

Angiography (also known as an *arteriogram*) is considered the most accurate test for coronary artery disease, because it shows definitely whether there's a blockage in the arteries, whereas other tests look at the *effects* of blockages. It is often used on women whose angina is worsening despite the use of medication (but microvascular angina cannot be effectively diagnosed with an angiogram).

Angiography can also be used to look for congenital abnormalities, valve problems or to evaluate patients for angioplasty or bypass surgery.

This is an invasive test, however, and it's not without risk. In rare cases, the procedure may cause a blood clot to form, and those patients may then have a heart attack or stroke. This is one reason why angiography is usually done in a hospital or in an outpatient facility attached to a hospital.

A patient may feel some pressure during the procedure and a momentary rush of heat, nausea or even a need to urinate when the dye is injected. After the procedure, the limb used for the catheter is kept at rest to avoid bleeding. If a leg artery or vein is used, temporary pressure may be applied until bleeding is controlled, and then the patient must keep her leg immobile for about four hours; activities should be limited for a day or two after the test. If an arm is used, the incision is stitched and the arm held in place and observed for eight to twenty-four hours.

While an angiogram is the most accurate test for establishing the degree of coronary artery disease, a controversial 1992 study in the *Journal of the American Medical Association* suggests that as many as half of all angiograms may not be medically necessary. The study found that when patients went for a second opinion as to whether they needed the test, 80 percent did not meet the study's criteria. So it might be wise to get another opinion if your doctor suggests an angiogram.

The decision whether or not to perform angiography (and the more aggressive therapies that may be recommended as a result) may be made on the basis of a patient's age, activity level and lifestyle, and the ultimate goal of treatment.

JEANNE'S STORY

"I had been having pretty bad angina for several months when they decided to do an angiogram.

"I asked the doctor to tell me what I was going to feel before I felt it so I wouldn't get nervous. They gave me a sedative and a local anesthetic where they put the catheter in my groin. It burned a little. My doctor told me about the dye feeling warm; he said, 'It's going to feel like you're in Florida.' I joked and said, 'No, it's more like the Bahamas.'

"The angiogram actually didn't hurt at all. You just feel some funny sensations, like this odd pressure moving inside your chest, or your heart palpitates. Afterward, I had to lie still for a long while and they had to push down on the incision—which was a little uncomfortable.

"What was interesting was that they have this TV screen, and you can see your arteries. They found two coronary blockages. They told me the blockages looked like they could be opened with a balloon catheter, and I could be put on medication. I was sort of relieved. When they told me it was something that could be treated, I just felt, well, I know I'm going to make it after all."

Magnetic Resonance Angiography (MRA): Now being tested as an alternative to angiography, *magnetic resonance angiography,* or MRA, uses the magnetic properties of body tissue to create an image. A person is placed within a magnetic resonance scanner, which is really a giant magnet, and radio waves are bounced off an area of the body. The radio waves bounce off different tissues in different ways, creating an image.

In this experimental form of magnetic resonance imaging, the blood is moving so fast through the blood vessels that it can't be seen but the vessel walls can be. If the blood isn't moving as fast as it should, it may mean there's a problem. Preliminary data suggests MR angiography may be almost as good as a conventional, but more invasive, angiogram.

NYU is testing special MRA machines that will image the coronary arteries in one tenth of a second, literally a "stop-motion" picture of the heart in mid-beat. It's hoped that MRA will eventually have an important place in cardiac diagnosis.

Once the various test results are evaluated and a diagnosis made, the next step is choosing an appropriate treatment.

13

Mending a "Broken" Heart

RECENT STUDIES HAVE shown that women are referred less often for invasive diagnostic tests, and receive less aggressive treatment. This is a complicated issue which we'll discuss in detail in Chapter 14. However, improvements in equipment and training have improved outcomes considerably, even for older women with more risk factors and health problems than their younger counterparts. So don't let fear or a physician's reluctance keep you away from potentially helpful treatments.

TREATING ANGINA

A woman with angina may receive one or more medications, depending on the frequency and severity of her symptoms. For *stable angina* (see page 179), drugs like nitroglycerine to dilate blood vessels, beta blockers to slow heart rate and calcium channel blockers to prevent blood vessel contraction may be prescribed, often in combination.

In 1994, new federal guidelines were issued for treating *unstable angina*. The condition causes severe and prolonged chest pains when a person is sleeping or at rest and affects more women than men. The new guidelines recommend use of aspirin as emergency treatment and say half of those diagnosed with unstable angina can be treated without hospitalization using medications such as anticlotting agents or blood thinners (including aspirin or heparin), as well as nitroglycerine or beta blockers. Calcium channel blockers are used if patients fail to respond to other medications. If drugs are ineffective, the guidelines call for angioplasty or other measures to restore blood flow in narrowed coronary arteries.

A major study of patients at forty-six hospitals in the United States and Canada found that aspirin can sometimes be as effective in controlling angina as clot-busting drugs or high-tech balloon angioplasty. (More about aspirin on page 221.)

Prinzmetal's or *variant angina* is also treated with nitrates, calcium channel blockers or beta blockers, which can curb artery spasms.

Angina patients may also suffer from hypertension and rapid heartbeats. In such cases, a combination of antianginal medications, antihypertension and antiarrhythmic drugs is needed, explains NYU cardiologist Sydney Mehl.

A woman with angina will be asked to make lifestyle changes including avoiding stress, emotional upsets and overexertion (especially after a big meal). Patients are usually asked to adopt a low-fat diet to slow the process of atherosclerosis (cholesterol-lowering drugs may also be needed), and to begin a regular regimen of moderate exercise. Stress-reduction exercises (see Chapter 8) also can be helpful. Of course, women who smoke will be advised to quit.

Antianginal drugs may have greater side effects in older women, since they tend to metabolize and excrete drugs more slowly. Physicians may choose to start the drugs at a lower dosage and increase the dose by smaller amounts in older women.

TYPES OF ANGINA MEDICATIONS

Nitroglycerine (Nitrates): Nitrates dilate the arteries so that blood can flow more freely through the heart. Nitroglycerine tablets (or timed-release capsules) are placed under the tongue at the first sign of an angina attack; they begin to work within five minutes. Nitroglycerine is also available as a mouth spray. Nitroglycerine's effects last between ten to fifteen minutes, and are used for relief of occasional angina symptoms.

For chronic angina, nitroglycerine can be given in longer-acting doses or a *skin patch* can deliver the medication continuously for up to eighteen hours. Twenty-four-hour use was found to cause a tolerance to the nitrate, however.

Potential Side Effects: Side effects can include severe headaches, dizziness, rapid heartbeat, flushing and low blood pressure, experienced as light-headedness when getting up from a bed or chair. Nitrates should not be taken with food.

Warning: Nitroglycerine may interact with antihypertensive medication, causing a sudden, severe drop in blood pressure. Skin patches need to be removed periodically (usually overnight) to prevent the development of tolerance to the drug.

Beta Blockers: Beta blockers such as propanolol (Inderal) or metoprolol (Lopressor) block the effects of chemicals, including adrenaline, produced during stress or exertion, which constrict blood vessels and boost the heart rate, increasing the heart's demand for oxygen. By lowering the heart rate and decreasing the strength of cardiac contractions, beta blockers prevent the oxygen deprivation to areas of the heart muscle that cause angina.

Potential Side Effects: Side effects include sluggishness and depression. Some women report difficulty achieving orgasm (some men suffer impotence). Beta blockers may worsen asthma, congestive heart failure and other conditions. They can also interact with anticlotting and cholesterol-lowering drugs.

Warning: In rare instances beta blockers can impair electrical rhythms in the heart, resulting in heart block. Doses must be carefully regulated. Anyone taking these drugs must be monitored by her physician.

Calcium Channel Blockers: In order for smooth muscle cells in our body to contract, including muscles in the heart and blood-vessel walls, calcium in the blood must combine with specific proteins inside muscle cells. Calcium channel blockers such as diltiazem (Cardizem CD), verapamil (Calan) and amiopidine besylate (Norvasc) prevent this process, improving blood flow to the heart. These drugs are also effective against angina caused by muscle spasm.

Potential Side Effects: Calcium channel blockers should be taken with milk or food to guard against possible stomach irritation and constipation. In people whose angina persists despite the use of other medications, calcium channel blockers may be prescribed with beta blockers and nitrates. Side effects may include dizziness, palpitations, fluid retention, headache, flushes and occasionally a rash.

Sources: *Physicians' Desk Reference, 1993; United States Pharmacopeia, Complete Drug Reference, 1993; Consumer Reports* books; Sydney J. Mehl, M.D., Clinical Assistant Professor of Medicine, NYU Medical Center.

If angina persists, despite medication and lifestyle changes, catheterization may be needed to widen narrowed arteries, using either of the following techniques:

Angioplasty: Balloon angioplasty involves the insertion into a blocked coronary artery of a thin plastic catheter with a miniature balloon at its tip. The catheter is threaded through a blood vessel in the groin or the arm until it reaches the site of a coronary blockage. The balloon is then inflated, flattening or cracking the plaque, slightly stretching the blood vessel.

In some cases, a tiny metal mesh scaffold called a *stent* is placed within the artery to keep it open. Stents may increase the risk of blood clots, because the endothelium, or cells lining coronary arteries, need to grow over the stent, and require a thin layer of clotting material to do this. The stent is usually covered within two to three weeks.

Studies show that women seem more prone than men to complications such as coronary-artery spasm, damage or artery collapse due to the pressure, causing a heart attack or prompting emergency bypass surgery. A 1993 report from the National Heart, Lung and Blood Institute found that women had a tenfold risk of dying in the hospital after undergoing angioplasty. However, over the long haul, other recent NHLBI data show that women do *just as well as men* after the procedure.

In about one third of all cases, the artery narrows again in three to six months. This is *not* due to reaccumulation of fatty deposits. Reclosure, or *restenosis*, is partly due to extra cell growth caused by the body's attempt to heal damage to the blood vessel lining during the procedure. If closure occurs, angioplasty can be repeated or a coronary bypass may be needed.

In 1994, the FDA approved the first stent to prevent restenosis in coronary arteries. The tiny stainless-steel device is folded like miniature scaffolding and threaded into the artery during balloon angioplasty, unfolding after the balloon is withdrawn. The cells lining the artery eventually grow over the stent. Patients receiving stents must take blood thinners for about a month, since clots can form on the stent while new tissue grows over it.

Atherectomy: In an atherectomy, a catheter equipped with a rotating cutting device shaves off and, in some cases, removes arterial plaques. One such catheter gathers the arterial debris to be removed in a small container attached to the cutting head.

The extent of the reopening of the coronary artery is assessed with an angiogram or intravascular ultrasound (see page 206). If the blockage is still severe, a balloon angioplasty can widen the artery further. Atherectomy can be effective in clearing obstructions at the beginning of arteries, and may be done after angioplasty has failed. However, it can damage artery walls and, if loose debris is left behind, may cause blockages in smaller blood vessels.

A 1993 report comparing atherectomy with balloon angioplasty in twelve hundred patients found that atherectomy was no better at clearing arteries or preventing them from narrowing again. The report, in the *New England Journal of Medicine*, also noted that atherectomy costs more and had more early complications. A number of recent studies have also found that the complication rate after atherectomy is more than three times greater among women. In general, however, atherectomy has been shown to be an effective procedure.

Laser Angioplasty: In 1992, the U.S. Food and Drug Administration approved the first laser angioplasty device, an Excimer laser, for patients who do not respond to balloon angioplasty. The device uses a fiber-optic catheter with a laser tip to melt away fatty plaques in coronary arteries.

The Excimer laser emits short bursts of ultraviolet light, generating heat that destroys the plaque, but dissipates before it can damage the artery wall. Balloon angioplasty may first be used to widen narrowed arteries sufficiently before inserting the laser tip.

Mark A. Adelman, M.D., an assistant professor of vascular surgery at NYU, cautions that, so far, lasers have *not* proven more effective than conventional angioplasty. In fact, he points out, the laser's thermal energy can stimulate atherosclerosis. Recent studies show that plaques seem to grow back faster on laser-treated areas than on those treated with balloon-tipped or atherectomy catheters. So it may be wise to avoid this procedure until it is perfected.

Experiments are now being conducted in Britain using ultrasound instead of lasers or balloons to break up blood clots.

Coronary Bypass Surgery: In cases of chronic, debilitating angina, if more than one coronary artery is dangerously narrowed by fatty plaques, or if the critical left-main artery is blocked, a coronary bypass may be needed.

A coronary bypass surgically grafts a healthy section of blood vessel to one or more areas of the heart, creating an alternate route for blood to nourish the heart with oxygen.

There are two types of bypass surgery. In a leg-vein graft, a vein is taken from the leg and sewn onto the blocked artery. An *internal mammary artery graft* (IMA) uses the thoracic artery inside the chest wall for the bypass. This artery is smaller in diameter than a leg vein, is thought to accumulate less atherosclerosis than leg veins and usually lasts longer.

IMA is a more technically difficult procedure, but studies show people receiving an IMA graft die less often following surgery in the hospital and have better long-term survival rates. At ten years, over 90 percent of mammary grafts are still open, compared with 50 percent of vein grafts.

Coronary artery bypass surgery takes about four hours to perform (longer for a mammary graft or a multiple bypass). Heart operations are usually done through an incision along the middle of the chest through the breastbone. During the surgery, a heart-lung machine takes over the work of pumping and purifying the patient's blood. (You might be able to donate your own blood to be used in the event a transfusion is needed; two to four pints are often needed. Blood cannot be predonated if patients have angina.)

After surgery, patients spend about two days in the postoperative cardiac intensive care unit, monitored around the clock. Within a week, most women can leave the hospital and recover at home.

About 80 percent of patients whose lives are being severely restricted by chronic angina will get considerable relief from their symptoms after a bypass. Women with the most blockages, who are most at risk for a heart attack, may gain years of life.

Complications from surgery can include heart attack and stroke, and the death rate during or after bypass surgery can be two to four times higher for women than for men. Moreover, a bypass is not a total *cure* for atherosclerosis. In most cases, grafted veins will begin to narrow with fatty plaques within five to seven years after the surgery if risk factors are not changed. Within ten years, 50 percent may become obstructed and another bypass may be needed. That picture may change in the future, however, as new surgical techniques emerge and new drugs are developed to keep blood vessels open longer after a bypass.

PEGGY'S STORY

"You would think that after you went through the [bypass] surgery and came through OK, you'd say, 'Let's go home and get on with life.' But even though I was feeling better physically, I kept feeling more de-pressed. One day, I started crying and just could not stop—I remember the nurse came and put a cool cloth on my face. The doctor came in and held my hand and reassured me that what I was going through was normal. The men find themselves crying too, he said. It's like hit-ting a brick wall: mortality. It's your first experience coming close to death. . . .

"After that, I started to get better. But it was months before I was my old cheerful self again."

TREATING HEART ATTACKS

Your survival after a heart attack can depend on a sequence of events that trauma-care experts call the "chain of survival."

The links in this chain consist of:

1. Early access: calling for and receiving prompt emergency medical help.

2. Early CPR (cardiopulmonary resuscitation) if needed.

3. Early defibrillation in the event of a dangerous heart rhythm dis-turbance during or just after a heart attack.

4. Early advanced care, getting state-of-the art coronary care, like clot-busting drugs.

The first link in the chain depends largely on your taking *immediate action* to get help if you are having symptoms of a heart attack. The second link, early CPR, can also depend on you or a family member knowing how and when to perform this lifesaving technique. In cardiac arrest, blood supply to the brain as well as to the heart is cut off after the heart stops pumping blood. If circulation is not restored, the brain will begin to die; studies show that adults have the best chance of surviving cardiac arrest if CPR was given within four minutes, and advanced life support within eight minutes. In fact, a 1991 study from Brown University said that if patients were not adequately revived at the scene (with CPR or defibrillation), they did not survive even after they were taken to the hospital. So speed in getting help is vital. CPR training takes about four hours and is available at low cost from your local Red Cross.

Once an ambulance arrives, a woman suffering a heart attack will probably be given oxygen through a face mask or nasal tubes to enhance the oxygen content of the blood still circulating to the heart. She may also be given an injection of morphine to relieve pain and anxiety; and her heartbeat will be monitored with an EKG to confirm that a heart attack is occurring (as well as to detect potentially deadly arrhythmias).

A coronary artery blockage can trigger chaotic rapid heartbeats or ineffectual fluttering of the muscles in the ventricles. When this occurs, blood collects in the heart. Immediate CPR, drugs or defibrillation are needed to restore blood flow and normal heart rhythm or sudden death can occur.

The third link in the chain of survival can depend on whether your local ambulance (or fire-emergency vehicle) is equipped with a portable defibrillator. The latest models use a computer to diagnose the nature of the arrhythmia en route to the hospital and to deliver the proper shock within milliseconds to restore a normal heart rhythm.

Upon your arrival at the emergency room, a blood test will be given to detect the presence of enzymes produced by damaged and dying heart cells. A new type of enzyme test was recently shown to be 95 percent accurate in determining if a person has had a heart attack, providing results in less than two hours.

The fourth link in the chain of survival, early advanced care, depends on the quality of the cardiac facility and the use of *thrombolytic agents*, drugs that help dissolve blood clots blocking the coronary artery before permanent damage is done to the heart. They are administered intravenously or are injected through a catheter into the affected coronary artery.

In 1994, the National Heart, Lung and Blood Institute issued new guide-lines recommending that heart attack patients receive clot-busting drugs within thirty minutes of their arrival at an emergency room. Some studies say that fewer than 40 percent of patients now receive clot-busting drugs.

The guidelines noted that a patient's medical history, such as a history of bleeding ulcers, may prohibit their use, since thrombolytics can cause dangerous bleeding from ulcers or even in the brain. Some research sug-gests women suffer bleeding complications and strokes after clot-busting therapy more often than men, but it's unclear why.

However, a 1994 study of more than 214,000 patients at 891 hospitals found that women who received thrombolytic therapy (such as t-PA) after a heart attack are much less likely to die than men.

The three major thrombolytic drugs in use today are: *streptokinase, urokinase* and *tissue plasminogen activator* (t-PA). The first two are enzymes that help break up blood clots; t-PA is genetically engineered from a human protein that dissolves clots. Heparin or aspirin may be given along with thrombolytics. Aspirin prevents platelets from sticking together to form new clots; heparin affects the proteins of clotting. Some patients who receive clot busters (either in the ambulance or emergency room) may undergo cardiac catheterization within twenty-four hours to make sure the clot is dissolved.

The results of a major study involving more than forty-one thousand heart attack patients in sixteen countries found that t-PA given with heparin was slightly more effective than heparin given with streptokinase. The 1993 report said that t-PA was *most* effective given within thirty minutes of a heart attack. Patients given a rapid injection of t-PA and heparin had 14 percent fewer subsequent heart attack deaths within thirty days. However, there was a slightly higher risk of stroke due to bleeding in the brain.

Another large international study found that taking aspirin immedi-ately after an attack, with or without clot-busting drugs, reduced the chances of suffering a second, nonfatal attack by 44 percent and the risk of having a fatal heart attack by 21 percent. (Aspirin also reduced the risk of blood clots after angioplasty and bypass surgery; death rates from heart attack are reduced threefold for two years after the procedures.)

A major difference between these drugs is cost. Giving aspirin right after a heart attack and for thirty days afterward costs about $13, com-pared with $320 for one dose of streptokinase and $2,300 for a single dose of t-PA.

In some locations in this country and Europe, thrombolytics are being administered in ambulances. The ongoing Myocardial Infarction Triage and Intervention (MITI) study in Seattle found that 40 percent of appropriately selected patients given clot busters en route to the hospital had little, if any, damage from their heart attacks.

ASPIRIN AND YOUR HEART

Some headline-making studies suggest that a low dose of aspirin every other day might keep coronary heart disease at bay in healthy people. There's no proof yet that this is true. *But there is definite, clinical evidence that aspirin does help women with heart problems.*

The best information comes from a major international study published in *The British Medical Journal* in 1994, which analyzed data from 300 studies involving 140,000 patients who were prescribed aspirin for heart attacks, strokes and other circulatory disorders. The "meta analysis" found that aspirin given to women after a heart attack reduced their risk of having a second attack by 25 percent. Aspirin was also found to save lives among women experiencing heart attacks and women who have survived strokes, even if they had a history of diabetes or high blood pressure.

Other studies show that a standard (325-milligram) aspirin tablet daily can reduce the risk of stroke in women who have had transient ischemic attacks (TIAs). Aspirin also reduces the likelihood of heart attacks in people with stable angina; it lessens symptoms and lowers the risk of heart attacks in patients with unstable angina; and it can decrease the chance of blood clots after angioplasty and bypass surgery.

For healthy women, however, there is no direct clinical evidence that aspirin will prevent coronary disease, stresses Julie E. Buring, Sc.D., principal investigator of the new Women's Health Study (WHS) at Harvard. The only data on aspirin and healthy women come from the Nurses' Health Study, which is based on questionnaires and is not a randomized clinical trial. It found that women who chose to take one to six 325-milligram aspirin tablets per week had a 25 percent lower risk of coronary disease; women over age fifty had a 32 percent lower risk. No benefits were found in taking more than six aspirin a week.

Dr. Buring says that clinical recommendations for healthy women taking aspirin to prevent heart attacks must wait for results of the WHS randomized prevention trial of low-dose aspirin (100 milligrams) taken every other day. The trial will last at least five years.

Aspirin's long-term effects in women are uncertain. Since aspirin interferes with clotting, it can increase the risk of strokes caused by bleeding into the brain. In high doses, aspirin can cause ulcers, gastro-intestinal bleeding, ringing in the ears and temporary hearing loss, among other things. The WHS will determine how these risks stack up against the potential benefits for healthy women.

For now, do not take aspirin on a regular basis without first consulting your doctor. Dr. Buring also stresses that taking aspirin is *not* a substitute for taking action on known cardiac risk factors, such as smoking, elevated blood cholesterol and high blood pressure.

In addition to anticlotting agents, beta blockers may be given in the hours following a heart attack, during recovery, and after a patient is sent home. Beta blockers reduce the heart rate by blocking the effects of chemicals like adrenaline produced during stress. They may also reduce anxiety in some patients, and they've been shown to reduce both the death rate and the chance of suffering a second heart attack by about 25 percent.

ACE inhibitors may also be used. These drugs block production of an enzyme that constricts the smooth muscle in blood vessel walls, lowering blood pressure and the strain on an already weakened heart, and may also prevent heart enlargement and second heart attacks.

Saving the Heart: The severity of a heart attack depends on which areas are affected and on whether dangerous arrhythmias occur during or after the attack. Critical areas of the heart include the left-main artery and the left anterior descending branch of that artery. If blood supply is cut off even briefly to the papillary muscle, which controls the heart valve, it can be deadly. The severity of heart damage can also depend on the effectiveness of *collateral circulation,* microscopic blood vessels that open and grow in people whose major arteries have become narrowed. These tiny blood vessels can provide a natural bypass for blood flow to the heart. Some women with heart disease develop more effective collateral circulation—an advantage if other avenues of blood supply are cut off.

Emergency balloon angioplasty may be performed to open blocked arteries in critical locations. This is risky, since the heart is vulnerable after an attack, and women often suffer complications from angioplasty under the best of circumstances. However, studies reported in 1993 suggest that balloon angioplasty can cut the risk of death and new heart attacks by as much as half.

If two or more blood vessels supplying the heart are blocked, an emergency bypass operation may be performed. For patients showing signs of heart failure, a balloon-tipped catheter may be rhythmically inflated to help push blood through the aorta and out to the body, almost like an auxiliary pump.

Depending on the severity of the attack, you will spend at least two to three days in the coronary care unit (CCU) of the hospital until doctors feel you're out of danger. There you'll be monitored twenty-four hours a day by a specially trained team of doctors and nurses. A bedside monitor will keep tabs on your heartbeat to spot potentially dangerous arrhythmias.

If chest pain persists, it could be a sign that heart cells are still dying or at risk of dying, and you may be given drugs like ACE inhibitors to relax the blood vessel walls, so that oxygen-rich blood can flow more freely to the heart.

Depending on your progress, you'll be moved to a regular hospital room or a cooperative care facility, if available. If necessary, you might be sent to an in-patient cardiac rehabilitation program (see page 140). When you're ready to go home, you'll be given exercises, guidelines on stress management, and a special diet. Medications may be prescribed for long-term use, and you need to know what each drug does and what the possible side effects may be in women.

PATRICIA'S STORY

"The hardest part for me was when I was about to go home from the hospital after my heart attack. You want to go home, but you're afraid to leave the doctors. You're depending on them to keep you alive. You're just filled with a lot of fears and emotions. I'm a widow and although my children are nearby, I was really worried: Who was going to take care of me now?"

BARBARA'S STORY

"I had a rough time dealing with the scars [from the bypass]. I wasn't so much worried about another heart attack—but the scars made me feel damaged. I worried: Would my husband still think I was attractive? But you know what he did? Some nights, he would gently massage the scars with some skin lotion. It was so sweet. More than anything, that made me feel like a whole woman again."

EMOTIONAL RECOVERY

The new American Heart Association Statement on Cardiovascular Disease in Women notes that women often have more depression, anxiety and guilt feelings about their illnesses than men. There may be a number of reasons for this.

Women are used to being caretakers; it may be hard for some women to adjust to needing to be taken care of by others. Since women are usually older when they suffer a heart attack, they're also more likely to be widowed or with grown children living far away. (It's estimated that three out of five American women over the age of sixty-five live alone, many in poverty.) Simple tasks like preparing a meal or making a bed may be daunting for a woman who's alone, still recovering and afraid of having another heart attack. Even if a woman is surrounded by family, her spouse or child may have difficulty assuming a temporary caretaker role, or may become overprotective. A woman may be fearful of becoming dependent on others.

"After a heart attack, a woman may be grieving her loss of autonomy. She may need to move in with her children or she may need home care. She is suddenly being confronted with limitations as well as the financial burden of recovery. And she fears being seen as an invalid in the eyes of her children and family," explains Sabina Primack, M.S.W, social-work supervisor for Cardiac Surgery at NYU Medical Center.

"How a woman deals with these feelings does impact on recovery and how functional she will become. Patients who receive counseling have less difficulty recovering and less postsurgical depression," Primack adds.

Counseling by a hospital social worker can help a woman prepare for the recovery process and any limitations she may face. Actively engaging in problem-solving and planning gives more of a sense of control. Preventing depression may also help a woman live longer. A 1993 study showed that people who survived heart attacks but suffered major depression had a three to four times' greater risk of dying in six months, compared to those who were not depressed.

How a woman perceives her recovery can also affect quality of life. Studies show that women who work outside the home take longer to return to their jobs, compared to men (despite resuming heavy-duty housework earlier). For many older women, much of their identity and self-esteem may be tied to taking care of their family; some women may not feel they've recovered completely unless they can do everything just as before.

A 1992 study from suburban California followed more than thirteen hundred men and women for over fifteen to twenty years after coronary bypass surgery, giving them yearly questionnaires on quality-of-life issues. Women consistently reported less satisfactory quality of life than men, notes Joseph S. Carey, M.D., a clinical associate professor of surgery at UCLA, who conducted the study at nearby Torrance Memorial Medical Center.

"Apparently men were more likely to take it easy after a heart attack, often retiring and enjoying a more leisurely lifestyle. The women, it seems, tried to return to their usual workload and found they couldn't. They couldn't do the laundry without getting short of breath, so they felt like they hadn't recovered as much as they should have. While the men, who were taking it easy, perceived themselves as feeling better," speculates Dr. Carey.

Just as men do, women need to take it slow and easy physically after a heart attack. A hospital social worker can work out care arrangements with family members or affordable home care for women who live alone.

Some women may have feelings of unattractiveness and (like many men) a fear that making love will bring on another heart attack. Scars from surgery may compound this feeling of undesirability. There's often a decrease in sexual activity after the initial recovery period, more from fear than from any physical limitations.

"The issue of sex is too often neglected among women," says Esther Chachkes, M.S.W., director of social work at NYU. "It's often assumed that older women are not as interested in this issue. That is not true. However, an older woman may be less comfortable *discussing* the subject. It should be discussed while planning cardiac rehabilitation."

A 1993 report found that the relative risk of a heart attack after sex among women (and men) who've had a prior attack is usually no greater than for healthy people. (Experts also say that sex won't damage bypass surgery.)

Some heart medications *can* interfere with sexual desire or functioning; don't be embarrassed to report any problems to your physician. Often a change in medication can resolve the problem.

Experts say sexual activity may generally be resumed two to three weeks after hospital discharge. But how do you know when you're ready physically? During lovemaking, your heart typically beats about one hundred and thirty times a minute, a little over the rate it reaches when you climb stairs. If you can climb stairs without your heart going twenty to thirty beats over its normal resting rate, and without shortness of breath or chest pain, you are probably physically ready to make love.

But if you don't feel ready, tell your partner. By the way, one Harvard study found recovering heart patients who were sexually active had a reduced risk of future heart attacks. In other words, a little loving will do your heart a world of good!

TREATING CARDIAC ARRHYTHMIAS

A number of drugs can be used singly or in combination to control irregular heartbeats, depending on the type of irregular beat. For example, in atrial fibrillation, the upper chambers of the heart beat wildly, up to three hundred beats per minute, and the lower chambers respond with irregular beats, so blood flow slows down and clots may form. Antiarrhythmic drugs are given to convert the atrial fibrillation to a normal or sinus rhythm, and anticoagulants are used to reduce the risk of clots, says NYU cardiologist Larry Chinitz, who specializes in the diagnosis and treatment of cardiac arrhythmias.

One drug, lidocaine, is a potent local anesthetic and is injected to control arrhythmias occurring after a heart attack or during heart surgery.

If another disorder is causing the arrhythmia, such as a thyroid abnormality, medication to treat the underlying problem may restore normal rhythm.

TYPES OF ANTIARRHYTHMIC DRUGS

Antiarrhythmic Drugs: Antiarrhythmic drugs such as digitalis slow the speed at which electrical impulses are conducted through the atrio-ventricular node and also slow contractions of the ventricles. Digoxin, a form of digitalis, slows the electric conductivity of the heart. Flecainide (Tambocor) slows nerve impulses in the heart, and makes heart tissue less sensitive.

Beta Blockers: These drugs suppress the effects of hormones that increase heart rate. They also enhance the effectiveness of antiarrhythmic drugs.

Calcium Channel Blockers: As they inhibit the flow of calcium in and out of cells, these drugs curb excess muscle contractions and slow the speed of electrical conduction in the heart. One of the most potent antiarrhythmics, amiodarone hydrochloride (Cordarone), acts as a beta blocker, alpha blocker (reducing the action of the stress hormone norepinephrine) and as a calcium channel blocker.

Potential Side Effects: Side effects can include dizziness, nausea, vomiting, constipation or diarrhea, indigestion, blurred vision, glaucoma, headaches, fatigue, insomnia, tremors, palpitations and, in rare cases, heart failure. Patients taking antiarrhythmic drugs may need to avoid coffee, tea, chocolate and aspirin compounds containing caffeine.

Warning: In 5 to 10 percent of patients, antiarrhythmic drugs may worsen their condition. The drug amiodarone may cause lung and liver inflammation as well as thyroid underactivity, muscle degeneration, slow heart rate and loss of balance. The antiarrhythmic procainamide (Procan SR) may lead to liver inflammation and prolonged use may cause lupus. Digoxin can be toxic in higher doses, and patients require monitoring. The drug flecainide is not used in patients with congestive heart failure or who have suffered a heart attack.

Sources: *Physicians' Desk Reference, 1993; United States Pharmacopeia, Complete Drug Reference, 1993; Consumer Reports* books; Larry A. Chinitz, M.D., Director, Cardiac Electrophysiology, NYU Medical Center.

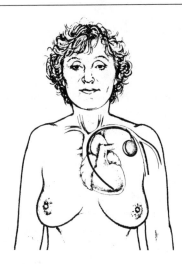

The pulse generator is surgically implanted in a pocket
of skin in the upper chest (for easy access in replacing batteries every eight to ten
years), and the wire leads are threaded through a nearby vein to the
appropriate chamber(s) of the heart. The lead wire delivers an electrical
impulse, causing the heart to contract. In dual-chamber pacemakers, the atrial
lead paces first, followed a fraction of a second later by the ventricular lead.
(Sources: National Institutes of Health; Dr. Larry Chinitz)

Pacemakers: With today's advanced technology and improvements in implantation surgery, a pacemaker may be preferable to drugs, says Dr. Chinitz. It can be used to control abnormally slow or rapid heartbeats and to treat heart block (a life-threatening interruption of electrical signals in the heart).

Today's "rate-adaptive" pacemakers can sense changes in movement, breathing or blood temperature. Their tiny computers are programmed to adjust the heart rate according to the level of activity.

Pacemaker implantation can be done in a cardiac catheterization lab, under local anesthesia. Patients may remain in the hospital for two to three days to make sure the device is working properly, and can resume normal activities (including sex) after two weeks. More strenuous activities, such as sports or heavy housework, are prohibited for two months to allow the wire leads to become firmly attached to the heart wall.

These days pacemakers can be checked periodically using a special transmitter that can send an electrocardiogram and a record of the pace-maker's rate to a physician over the telephone.

Implantable Defibrillators: These devices are now being used to treat dangerously rapid heartbeats that can cause sudden death, especially if a patient has suffered a heart attack. They are miniature versions of the electric generator and paddles used to restore a heartbeat after cardiac arrest.

A pulse generator about the size of a pack of cards is surgically implanted in a pocket of skin on one side of the abdomen, and a tiny wire (or pole) is placed in the right ventricle and connected to this power source. When the leads detect a dangerously rapid heartbeat, electrode patches on the heart (or additional wires in the heart) will deliver a small electric shock to restore the normal rhythm of the heart.

"The new generation of defibrillators eliminate the patch and allow implantation of the device solely through a single wire and an active 'battery can' implanted in the chest like a pacemaker, which will not only generate a pulse but act as a pole of the defibrillation unit," explains Dr. Chinitz.

Defibrillators can treat very slow heartbeats by acting as a backup pacemaker until the heart resumes its normal function. They also can communicate with computers, so physicians can monitor the activity of the defibrillator and the patient.

The recovery period following implantation is similar to that of a pacemaker, with gradual resumption of physical activities, along with a series of diagnostic tests to make sure the device is working properly.

Dr. Chinitz cautions that there is a slight risk of fainting during defibrillation, so patients may have some lifestyle limitations and may not be able to drive or operate heavy machinery. For most people, however, the benefits outweigh the restrictions. Studies show that the devices allow severely ill patients to live an average of ten years longer.

Cardioversion: If chronic arrhythmias are not helped by drugs or if there is a life-threatening arrhythmia (such as ventricular fibrillation after a heart attack), an electric shock may be given to jolt the heart back to its normal rhythm. This is called *cardioversion.*

The electric current is sent to the heart from a defibrillator through conduction paddles placed on the chest (as with an EKG, a conduction gel is used). The current stuns the heart cells for an instant, allowing the sinus node to reestablish a normal rhythm.

Radiowave Ablation: Sometimes disease or birth defects leave an abnormal area of heart cells that interfere with the heart's electrical impulses, causing rapid heartbeats. A new treatment for this type of tachycardia involves cardiac catheterization and high-frequency radio waves.

A catheter is threaded through a vein to the problem area of the heart. Radio frequency current (similar to microwaves) fed through the catheter generates heat in the heart tissue, scarring the tiny clutch of abnormal cells. The procedure is done under mild sedation and local anesthesia in a cardiac cath lab, and produces little or no discomfort.

One note: survivors of ventricular tachycardia or ventricular fibrillation are advised not to drive for at least one month (possibly as long as seven months) after being discharged from the hospital. Experts say recurrent arrhythmias could affect driving ability.

TREATING HEART FAILURE

If inadequate heart-muscle contraction or a valve problem is causing the heart to pump ineffectively, the diagnosis is usually heart failure. Because not enough blood is being pumped from the heart, pressure builds up in the veins and fluids accumulate, or congest, in body tissues (which is why the condition is often referred to as *congestive heart failure*).

To correct these problems, the first thing usually prescribed is rest and a low-salt diet. Digitalis is often given to strengthen the heart's contractions so more blood can be pumped and less congestion occurs, says NYU cardiologist Sydney Mehl.

"Diuretics may be prescribed to help get rid of excess fluid in body tissues and reduce blood volume, so the left chamber doesn't become enlarged and the heart doesn't have to work harder," he explains.

New guidelines issued by the U.S. Department of Health and Human Services recommend more aggressive use of ACE inhibitors, which relax blood vessels, help the heart pump more effectively and slow deterioration of heart muscle. Other medications include vasodilators, which open smaller blood vessels, reducing resistance to blood flow, and calcium channel blockers, which may also help dilate blood vessels. If heart failure is being caused by high blood pressure, antihypertensive medication may be used. If the cause is a damaged or narrowed valve, surgery may be needed to repair or replace the valve.

The 1994 guidelines urge patients to seriously follow advice to stick to low-salt diets and take all medications prescribed, monitor daily weight gain (from fluid retention) and exercise.

TYPES OF HEART-FAILURE DRUGS

Digitalis: Derived from the foxglove plant, digitalis has been in use for more than two hundred years. Digitalis drugs (digoxin or digitoxin) allow more calcium to enter heart-muscle cells and enhance the force of the heart's contractions; the heart then pumps more blood, reducing the tendency to retain fluid and preventing the heart from becoming enlarged due to overwork. Digoxin also slows the heart rate, so the heart can beat more effectively. These drugs may be combined with diuretics and ACE inhibitors.

Potential Side Effects: Side effects can include fatigue, weakness, headaches, nausea, vomiting, loss of appetite, irregular or slowed heart rhythm and vision disturbances.

Warning: Digitalis compounds frequently interact with other medications and can build to toxic levels in the blood, so patients need to be carefully monitored.

Sources: *Physicians' Desk Reference, 1993; United States Pharmacopeia, Complete Drug Reference, 1993; Consumer Reports* books; Sydney J. Mehl, M.D., Clinical Assistant Professor of Medicine, NYU Medical Center.

Heart Transplant: If the heart is so damaged that it does not respond to therapy or surgery, a heart transplant is the treatment of last resort. Occasionally, both the heart and lungs are transplanted.

More than two thousand transplants are performed every year, mostly on men. Donors must be carefully matched for blood type and heart size, and the cause of death must not have harmed the heart.

The average age of a female transplant recipient is thirty-nine (for men, it's forty-seven). Patients have a 72 percent chance of surviving for five years after a transplant, staying on an appropriate combination of medications. Since complications can include rejection of the transplant by the body's immune system, drugs are given to suppress these immune reactions.

Patients with end-stage heart failure may be given a *left ventricular-assist device (LVAD)*, to help a diseased heart function while a donor heart can be found. The LVAD consists of a pumping chamber, about six inches in diameter, implanted in the abdomen and connected to the heart across the diaphragm. Its electric-powered pump collects blood from the left ventricle and ejects it into the aorta, as a healthy heart would.

Alternatives to heart transplants are also being explored, including a new treatment regimen using new combinations and doses of existing medications to relax blood vessels and allow more blood to flow through the heart. Studies show such regimens allow more than half of patients with severe heart failure to function as well, and live just as long, without a heart transplant.

TREATING STROKES

Transient ischemic attacks (TIAs) and ischemic strokes are often treated with anticoagulants, which interfere with blood-clotting factors (such as warfarin or heparin) and/or small daily doses of aspirin, which inhibit platelets from gathering into clots. A drug called ticlopidine (Ticlid) is sometimes prescribed for people who can't take aspirin, or if aspirin doesn't work.

Approximately 15 to 20 percent of strokes are directly caused by a severe narrowing of the carotid artery, which supplies blood to the brain. This may be helped by surgery, called *carotid endarterectomy*, which involves making an incision in the neck, clamping the artery involved, and opening it to remove the debris (a shunt is put around the clamp to maintain blood flow to the brain). Afterward, the artery is stitched closed and, if it is badly damaged, repaired with a Dacron patch.

A 1994 study conducted at thirty-nine medical centers in the United States and Canada found that carotid endarterectomy can cut the risk of ischemic stroke by half over a five-year period. However, the study of 1,662 people found that the surgery was less beneficial for women, with a risk reduction of 16 percent, compared to 69 percent for men. Further studies are needed to find out why.

The surgery is most helpful for patients whose carotids are more than 70 percent blocked, and who experience temporary stroke symptoms, such as blindness in one eye, loss of speech and brief weakness in one side of the body. Studies are under way to see if the surgery will help people with less severe blockages.

Therapy for TIAs and ischemic strokes also includes modification of risk factors such as smoking, and controlling hypertension and diabetes.

For acute stroke, a patient is first stabilized to maintain blood pressure and fluid balance, and to minimize secondary complications such as pneumonia and paralysis. Carotid endarterectomy may help prevent further brain damage. If there has been impairment from a stroke, a rehabilitation program will be needed to help restore as much speech and mobility as possible.

Today, many major strokes—and deaths from stroke—are being prevented by aggressive treatment of hypertension, and the careful monitoring and treatment of women who suffer TIAs.

14

Getting the Best Medical Care

EVEN THOUGH JUST as many women die of heart attacks as men, up until fairly recently the scientific community has regarded coronary heart disease as strictly a male affliction. Of the more than two hundred clinical trials on heart disease treatments over the past thirty years, fewer than 20 percent of the research subjects were women. A majority of the trials also excluded people over age seventy-five, even though older heart patients are more likely to be female. As a result, no specific diagnostic criteria exist for women, nor is there information on how treatments may interact with a woman's unique physical and biochemical factors.

Moreover, many recent studies have uncovered an apparent pattern of gender bias in how women are treated for heart disease. The questions are now being asked: Why are women treated differently? How has it affected their outcomes? And what can women *do* about it?

MARIE'S STORY

"I was a teacher for twenty-five years; I'm retired now. Eight years ago, I was especially stressed at school and began having chest pains. My doctor did an EKG but found nothing. He told me I had no reason to worry; it was probably just emotional anxiety or even menopause.

"But I would still have these frequent twinges and pressure in my

234

chest. I would stop whatever I was doing, and they would go away. But since the doctor didn't seem concerned, I wasn't, either. This year, I had a small heart attack and underwent a bypass.

"My doctor had it in his records that both my parents had suffered heart attacks and that my brother had a stroke. But he never put two and two together.

"They say women are ignored or forgotten in heart disease. But I think it's partly because women basically stay healthier until menopause and after that, it comes on very fast.

"I'd like to see more education of family physicians about heart disease and women, because they're our first line of defense against this disease."

HOW BEING FEMALE
MAY AFFECT MEDICAL CARE

Four major studies indicate that sex differences in the diagnosis and treatment of heart disease may begin when a woman reports the very first symptoms of chest pain to her doctor.

Researchers at the Albert Einstein College of Medicine in New York first reported in 1987 that doctors were more than three times as likely to dismiss a woman's complaints of chest pain as "psychiatric." A 1990 report in the *Journal of the American Medical Association* said men were *seven times* more likely to be referred for cardiac arteriography after complaining of chest pain, whereas women's chest pain was more likely to be written off as stress, anxiety or even heartburn. A 1991 study in the *Annals of Internal Medicine* concluded that women have to be significantly sicker than men to get prompt treatment for their cardiac symptoms. And a 1994 study from St. Louis University in the *Annals* found that among a group of 3,975 men and women ages forty-five to sixty-five with suspected coronary disease referred for an exercise stress test, women with positive test results were *half as likely* to be referred for further evaluation as men who had identical risk factors, symptoms and positive test results. Twice as many men underwent angioplasty or other revascularization procedures, while three times as many women died during two years of follow-up.

Why should this happen? Nina Bickell, M.D., M.P.H., a former assistant professor of clinical medicine at NYU who has extensively studied the issue of gender bias, points out that a doctor makes a diagnosis based on how common a particular disease is in the patient's age and gender group. A forty-five-year-old woman complaining of chest pain is statistically less likely to have heart disease than a man of the same age, so physicians are less likely to consider it as a diagnosis. In fact, a small 1994 study by researchers at Duke University found that women were referred less often than men for cardiac catheterization because physicians predicted (in this case, accurately) that the women were less likely to have serious heart disease.

In addition, women often display atypical symptoms of angina, different from the classic chest pressure or pain radiating down the left arm usually reported by men. Test results may also be inconclusive in women, especially in younger women, says Dr. Bickell, now with the New York State Department of Health at Albany. The false positive rate for exercise stress tests is about one third in women; the false negative rate may be as high as 25 percent. It's theorized that women may have different physiologic responses to exercise than men, and their test results are less accurate when measured against a standard geared toward men. Women's breast tissue can also create a shadow that mimics a coronary blockage in a thallium stress test.

Although an angiogram is just as accurate for detecting problems in the heart and major blood vessels in women as it is in men, researchers at the National Heart, Lung and Blood Institute speculate that in some women, blockages may occur in blood vessels *too tiny* to be seen on a standard angiogram. So a woman may be referred to a gastroenterologist or a psychiatrist for her symptoms.

Even when an accurate diagnosis is made, a number of recent studies conclude that women with heart disease are treated less aggressively than men. A 1991 report in the *New England Journal of Medicine* found that among 2,231 patients with angina, *half* as many women were referred for cardiac catheterization or coronary bypass surgery, compared to men. Nationwide statistics from the American Heart Association bear this out; 107,000 women underwent angioplasty compared with 223,000 men; 296,000 men had bypass surgery, as opposed to 111,000 women.

A survey of patients treated for heart attacks at nineteen Seattle-area hospitals also showed clot-busting drugs were given to half as many women as men. The Seattle researchers speculate that women may have had less severe symptoms and delayed seeking medical care, or their heart attacks may have been masked by some other condition. Since clot busters only work within a few hours of a heart attack, a woman may have already missed this window of opportunity by the time she's diagnosed.

Some women may not receive equal care simply because they have no way to pay for it. The Jacobs Institute of Women's Health estimates 12 to 14 percent of women in this country presently have no health insurance, and the rates are even lower among black and Latina women. Single, separated, divorced or unemployed women are also more likely to be uninsured. All told, perhaps sixteen to seventeen million American women have severely limited access to medical care. Hopefully, this situation will change when universal health coverage is finally adopted.

Race and socioeconomic status may also determine who gets treatment. A recent report in the *Journal of the American Medical Association* found the percentage of black women who underwent coronary bypass surgery was less than half that for white women. Some possible explanations given were poverty, a reluctance to have surgery, racial prejudice among physicians and lack of medicaid copayment as contributing factors.

THE GENDER GAP IN OUTCOME

Even when women do get prompt diagnosis and treatment, they suffer more complications, derive less benefit from clot-busting drugs and die more often in the hospital than men.

A 1993 update from an ongoing NHLBI research project found that women are up to ten times more likely than men to die in the hospital after undergoing angioplasty. Even when the researchers adjusted for age and the severity of disease, the risk of death was more than four times greater for women.

Katherine Detre, M.D., Ph.D., a professor of epidemiology at the University of Pittsburgh and director of several gender studies for the National Heart, Lung and Blood Institute, notes that women are usually older and sicker when their heart disease comes to medical attention, and they tend to have a greater incidence of coexisting health problems.

Indeed, a study of more than ten thousand angioplasty patients at Emory University Hospital in Atlanta found that the women were an average of five years older than the men; 55 percent of the women were hypertensive, compared with 40 percent of the men; twice as many women as men had heart failure; and more women than men had diabetes.

The 1994 Emory study concluded that age and illness, not gender, accounted for the women's higher mortality. But other research shows that even when the health profiles of men and women are the *same*, gender differences in outcome persist.

For example, recent studies suggest that clot-busting drugs may not prevent deaths as well in women after a heart attack. A three-year study of more than thirty-three hundred male and female heart attack patients at Boston's Brigham and Women's Hospital revealed that when men and women received the thrombolytic t-PA (tissue plasminogen activator) within the first four hours after an attack, women were twice as likely to die as men. Six months to a year later, twice as many women as men had died. European studies also show that women do not get as much benefit as men from streptokinase (the chief alternative to t-PA).

Opinions vary as to what causes these deadly differences. One theory is that women's blood contains more fibrinogen (a key clotting substance), which may hamper the effectiveness of clot busters; women may need different doses of these drugs.

Other experts claim women's blood vessels are smaller, become blocked more easily and are harder to work with surgically. The Northern New England Cardiovascular Disease Study Group, based at the Dartmouth-Hitchcock Medical Center, has been studying angioplasty, bypass and heart-valve surgery in men and women since 1987. The study director, Gerald T. O'Connor, Ph.D., D.Sc., explains that the amount of body surface (calculated from height and weight) is used as an index to set the pump that circulates blood during open-heart surgery. Women typically have less body surface area than men, and the internal diameter of their coronary arteries can be 0.17 to 0.23 millimeters smaller than men's. It's a tiny difference, but one which Dr. O'Connor says can be important to blood flow during and after a bypass. His study team found that *both* women and men with a small body surface were four times more likely to die in the hospital after surgery. Body and blood-vessel size were also associated with increased risk of hemorrhage, heart failure and closure of the grafted blood vessel (the most common causes of death after surgery for women).

Dr. O'Connor also notes that more women than men are listed as emergency, or "urgent," patients and this can affect their care. Of the two types of bypass surgery—a leg-vein graft or an internal mammary artery (IMA) graft—the Dartmouth study found that women were less likely to receive an IMA graft, even though it has a lower incidence of in-hospital deaths and better long-term survival. An IMA graft is more difficult, since the vessels involved are smaller and less accessible than leg veins, and is far less likely to be done in an emergency. More women than men need emergency bypass surgery, and Dr. O'Connor suggests this may be why fewer women get an IMA graft.

Smaller artery diameter may also make angioplasty technically more difficult in women. For example, when the balloon at the end of the catheter is inflated to break away a coronary blockage, that's when women often experienced problems. In rare cases, the artery may collapse from the pressure, or the artery may go into uncontrollable spasms that cause it to collapse, triggering a heart attack or prompting an emergency bypass.

The picture may be improving with better equipment and training, stresses Sheryl F. Kelsey Ph.D., associate professor of epidemiology at the University of Pittsburgh and deputy director of the NHLBI angioplasty registry. "Women may have more complications due to a worse cardio-vascular risk profile," she comments. "But overall, the success rate and long-term prognosis after angioplasty are excellent, and women should not be denied these procedures."

In fact, studies show that once women make it past the critical post-surgery period, they do as well as men. A fifteen-year study by the University of Washington found *long-term survival after a bypass was virtually the same for men and women*. The NHLBI's data show similar long-term benefits for women after angioplasty.

"What's needed are studies comparing the outcomes of bypass and angioplasty *in women*, so we can determine the *true* risks and effectiveness in women and why," stresses Dr. Kelsey.

AS A WOMAN, FACTORS THAT MAY AFFECT YOUR CARE

- If you are over age sixty-five
- If you have high blood pressure
- If you have diabetes
- If you have unstable angina
- If you have a small body size (blood-vessel size is smaller)

ARE WOMEN BEING "MIS-TREATED"?

Are aggressive treatments like bypass surgery actually used less often in women because they may be older, sicker and have higher complication rates? Or are female heart patients being "mis-treated"?

A 1993 report in the *Journal of Women's Health* found that gender alone accounts for up to 25 percent of the differences in the care of men and women with heart disease. The authors conclude that diagnosis and treatment may still be influenced by "gender stereotypes and general conceptions about the nature of CHD (coronary heart disease) as a man's disease. . . . Even small effects of gender bias are of concern because inappropriate decisions in only 2 or 3 percent of cases can have life or death consequences for several thousand people."

NYU's Dr. Nina Bickell is trying to find out how treatment decisions are made and how they impact on female patients. Her first report, published in 1992, looked at the treatment given to 5,797 patients with coronary artery disease. Among the sickest patients, who had the most to gain in potential survival from a bypass, equal numbers of men and women were referred for bypass surgery. However, among patients at lowest risk for dying, more men than women were referred for a bypass.

One conclusion, says Dr. Bickell, is that if cheaper, less-invasive methods like medication relieve symptoms and improve survival as effectively as surgery, then the "gender bias" of fewer women receiving a bypass inadvertently resulted in more appropriate medical care for women—and more *unnecessary* surgery for men.

"However, if the quality of life is worse with medical treatment than with surgery, then more is being done to improve the quality of life for men," says Dr. Bickell. "If that turns out to be true, then women *are* being harmed."

At the same time, an editorial in the March 1993 edition of *Circulation* cautioned physicians against making treatment decisions to compensate for a perceived "gender gap":

"Until we learn more about how gender affects outcome, we have to make decisions based on what's currently known about risk," wrote Hiltrud S. Mueller, M.D., associate director of Cardiology at Montefiore Medical Center in New York, coauthor of the editorial. "In the end, if the risks are too great and a treatment will not make a patient feel better or live longer, the procedure should not be done."

However, Dr. Mueller and her coauthor believe that all the attention being paid to the issue of gender bias will result in more knowledge about heart disease in women and, ultimately, in better care.

JEANNE'S STORY

"You know what my biggest complaint is? Some doctors don't listen. They seem to act only if there's a crisis.

"Women tend to talk about emotional things, and doctors don't want to hear that; that's not how they were trained. Doctors are also too specialized; you go to a podiatrist, he doesn't look above the ankle. You have to see someone else about the pains in your leg. Some of them give you the idea they have no time to talk or that you don't have the brains to understand what they're saying. That offends me.

". . . I've learned to speak up and stand my ground when I think there's a problem. I tell.the doctor when I don't like something, and I question everything. You really have to."

COMMUNICATING WITH YOUR DOCTOR

A woman's biggest problem in cardiac care may be getting a doctor to take her—and her symptoms—seriously.

A survey on American Women's Health by the Commonwealth Fund found that 25 percent of women (compared with 12 percent of men) felt that their doctors talked down to them, and 17 percent (versus 7 percent of men) have been told that a medical complaint was "all in their head."

The American Medical Association admits such sexual stereotyping does occur. In their 1990 statement "Gender Disparities in Clinical Decision-Making," the AMA said: "Some evidence suggests physicians are more likely to attribute women's health complaints to emotional, rather than physical causes." The AMA said women's tendency to be more concerned about their health and to visit doctors more often than men is often seen, not as a positive trait, but as "overanxiousness" (read: *hypochondriac*).

In terms of cardiac care, the AMA speculated that since angina is more common in women, it may not be viewed as being as serious a symptom as it is in men. The statement added that perhaps more aggres-

eatment may be given to men because their social role is tradition-
,een as more valuable than women's. The AMA urged physicians to
amine their practices and attitudes for the influence of social or cultural biases that could affect medical care."

There are some important steps that you can take to overcome unconscious gender bias, and communicate more effectively with your
doctor:

• *First, write down your symptoms and health history in precise, non-
emotional terms.* Mack Lipkin, Jr., M.D., director of the Division of Primary Care and Internal Medicine at NYU-Bellevue Hospital Center and
president of the American Academy on Physician and Patient Studies,
says his studies of medical interviews reveal that women tend to describe
their symptoms in more emotional terms, whereas doctors are trained to
view symptoms in a purely clinical sense. Hence, a woman's chest pains
may be classified as "vague" or "emotional."

This idea was actually tested in a small trial by researchers at the
Oklahoma University Health Sciences Center. They randomly divided
forty-four mostly male physicians into three groups. Two groups saw vid-
eotapes of the same actress portraying a forty-year-old patient describing
symptoms of chest pain in two stereotyped styles. In one tape, the "patient" was emotional, dramatic and flamboyantly dressed; in the other,
she was businesslike and conservatively dressed. A third group read a
verbatim transcript of the "patient" describing her symptoms. In each
case, the patient's words were identical.

The researchers reported that 73 percent of the physicians who viewed
the "histrionic" patient made a *non*-cardiac diagnosis (mostly panic attacks or anxiety), while only 13 percent chose a cardiac diagnosis. Half
the physicians who viewed the businesslike presentation chose cardiac
diagnoses, and 93 percent recommended noninvasive testing (compared
with 53 percent of those who saw the emotional presentation). Their
conclusion: A woman's communication style *can* profoundly affect a physician's diagnostic approach.

• *Second, go prepared for your office visit with specific questions* (see below), especially if there is an existing medical problem. Be assertive in
asking questions and discussing *all* symptoms, even those that may seem
insignificant. Don't allow any doctor to dismiss a complaint as being "all
in your head." Let your doctor know about your health concerns, and
what you expect him or her to do for you.

• *Third, discuss the business of your health in a businesslike manner and setting.* Don't have lengthy discussions with your doctor while you're sitting half-naked on the examining-room table and feeling vulnerable; Dr. Lipkin advises women to get dressed and sit down in the doctor's office to talk on a more equal footing.

• *Fourth, bring a family member or friend to the doctor's office to aid in the communication process and to act as your advocate.* This is a good idea if you find it difficult to be assertive. A third party can also take notes and ask questions, especially if there is a language barrier, and can make communication easier for the physician as well.

• *Fifth, take notes.* Dr. Lipkin strongly recommends that women take a small tape recorder to doctor visits, especially those with specialists where treatment options are discussed. A physician shouldn't mind if you ask to tape a discussion; the tape can help you and your family review what was said later on. Ask your physician to translate medical jargon, and double-check all instructions.

• *Sixth, don't ever hesitate to get another opinion.* Symptoms of disease in an older woman may be seen by both doctor and patient as a normal part of aging. Coronary disease is *not* a "normal" part of aging.

• *Finally, if you are not satisfied with a physician's explanations or answers to your questions, ask again.* If a doctor doesn't seem to be listening or interrupts frequently, find a physician who will be more attentive. Medical care is a commodity, and you are paying for it.

TEN KEY QUESTIONS FOR YOUR DOCTOR

1. Which tests are being given and what are the alternatives, if any?
2. On what basis was a diagnosis made: tests, symptoms or an educated guess?
3. Why is a particular therapy being suggested and what is the doctor's own experience with the treatment?
4. How long will treatment take and how will it affect me?
5. Would another treatment be just as effective for my problem?
6. What will the costs be and what kind of facility will be used? What will I gain from going to a larger facility?
7. How long will recovery take and what are the possible problems I may encounter?

8. What drug is being prescribed (if any), what is it supposed to do and how is it taken? Are there any possible side effects I should be concerned about, or things I should watch for?

9. What happens if I miss a dose? When can I stop taking this medication?

10. Would your recommendations be the same for a man in my condition in the same situation?

Sources: The People's Medical Society; The National Council on Patient Information and Education; Mack Lipkin, M.D., NYU Medical Center; Jane Sherwood, R.N., M.S.N., Deaconess Hospital.

ANGELA'S STORY

"I am an actress by profession and I work as a health advocate within the Latino community in Ventura County and Los Angeles. Through my own illness a few years ago, I came to realize the depth of the problems unique to Latinos that so often prevent us from seeking and obtaining proper medical care.

"It is not just the Spanish language that makes us different. A host of unique cultural barriers pose equally difficult barriers. Secrecy, denial, a reluctance to question authority and a history of neglect at the hands of a system that does not comprehend our differences has resulted in a substandard level of care, suffering and mortality for Latinos.

"Our desire to protect our families from anything harmful and the acute sense of privacy that prevents open discussion of illness, even between spouses, also works to our disadvantage.

"In addition, our religious beliefs, so often a source of strength, can foster a sense of fatalism, in place of knowledge and personal control."

RACE, CULTURE AND YOUR HEALTH

Many Americans do not realize how bicultural they are and how strong their cultural beliefs may be, while many women want to maintain a strong ethnic or cultural identity. The latest census figures show women of color (including blacks, Latinas and Asians) make up more than one quarter of the American population.

While there are tremendous variations within large ethnic and cultural groups (such as Asians or Hispanics whose families originally came from different countries or regions), recent studies have shed light on some general hurdles to health care.

Studies show that due to historical factors, blacks and Hispanics often have a distrust of doctors (and a medical "system" that's not user-friendly in general), which may delay a woman's seeking care and may hamper communication with a doctor. Many Hispanic and Korean-American patients are reluctant to ask questions of their doctor or go for a second opinion because they believe it is challenging authority.

In addition, some religions and cultures have a fatalistic attitude, believing death is preordained or that illness is a punishment for past sins. Hindus or Buddhists believe that suffering is an inevitable part of life, so perhaps cardiac symptoms or side effects of treatment may be tolerated unnecessarily, rather than reported to a physician, says Marjorie Kagawa-Singer, Ph.D., M.N., R.N., a medical anthropologist and an associate researcher at the National Research Center for Asian American Mental Health in Los Angeles.

The Western concept of preventive medicine is a strong part of Asian health beliefs. The Chinese use herbs, acupuncture and exercise to maintain a balance of energy in the body, which they believe wards off disease. However, in Chinese culture, there is a superstition that one does not go looking for symptoms or signs of disease; to do so may bring about that event. For example, buying health insurance may be seen as "buying trouble."

Among some Asian groups, heart disease does not have the same cultural significance as in the West, observes Dr. Kagawa-Singer. In Chinese and Japanese cultures, the soul is thought to reside in the belly, so diseases of the abdominal area may provoke greater concern.

Many groups believe that blood is sacred and cannot be replaced once it is removed from the body, so they avoid surgery or blood tests. Christian Scientists and Jehovah's Witnesses have deep religious beliefs that often clash with established medical practices and technology, as do Pentecostal Protestant sects within the Latino community.

Many ethnic groups use their own herbal medicines, alternative health providers (such as herbalists or *spiritistas*), and treatments (like acupuncture), in addition to Western medical treatments. Too often physicians have dismissed such practices, so women are hesitant to tell their doctor they are using them.

Doctors are now becoming more aware of such cultural factors. What *you* can do is try to help your physician understand *your* particular feelings and beliefs, as well as fears you may have picked up about an illness during childhood.

Discuss *all* aspects of your treatment, including other therapies you may be trying in addition to what's been prescribed. Remedies like herbal teas, for example, can interact with prescription drugs.

If something is a potential problem, deal with it openly. Admittedly, this is often very difficult to do. But you need to make your views and your needs known in order to be an active participant in your health care.

FINDING THE RIGHT PHYSICIAN

Among the most important things you can do is *not* to confine your medical care to the gynecologist. The American College of Obstetricians and Gynecologists reports that over half of all American women regard their OB-GYN as their principal physician. Consequently, OB-GYNs must deal with a host of medical problems beyond their specialized training in the female reproductive system.

If you're nearing menopause or past it, find a good primary-care physician, an internist who is aware of women's special risks of heart disease (ask about this issue when "interviewing" a doctor you're considering), one who will be attentive to your general health concerns.

Make sure the physician or surgeon you choose is board-certified or accredited in his or her specialty. If you need a cardiologist, seek one who has been board-certified by the American College of Cardiology. To earn a fellowship in the American College of Cardiology, a doctor must devote three years of study specifically to heart disease and must pass a series of tough exams. Only then can the coveted initials *F.A.C.C.* appear after the *M.D.* You also want to look for someone affiliated with a teaching hospital or medical center with a strong, respected cardiology department.

Credentials aside, you also want to pick a doctor with whom you can develop a good working relationship. This is where recommendations and insights from a friend can help.

As part of every office visit, a good physician should make time to talk with patients about their general health and any problems or symptoms they may be experiencing. You should be comfortable enough with your doctor to talk about any facet of your life, however intimate, that could be affecting your health.

Many women feel a female physician will be more empathetic. And indeed, Dr. Lipkin's research has found that women doctors conduct longer office visits, give more detailed information than male physicians and actively build positive partnerships with patients. (A recent study in the *New England Journal of Medicine*, which looked at the patient records of almost ninety-eight thousand women in Minnesota, found that those who received their care from female physicians were twice as likely to receive a Pap smear, and 40 percent more likely to receive a mammogram.)

Often, however, a woman physician's views on treatment are surprisingly not that different from those of her male counterparts. Your choice of a physician should not depend on gender alone.

Some women feel that a physician who is a member of their racial or ethnic group may be more appreciative of cultural differences and more able to bridge language barriers. Feeling comfortable with a physician is extremely important, but so is picking the best doctor.

If you are a member of a health maintenance organization (HMO) or other managed care plan and you are not happy with a doctor, ask for a list of other physicians within the group.

HOW TO FIND A GOOD DOCTOR

If you're looking for a primary-care physician, you can start with your local medical center or medical school. The American Society of Internal Medicine can provide you with a list of board-certified internists in your area.

If you have the name of a physician you're considering, you can write to the American Medical Association for a physician profile, which gives the details of a doctor's training and specialties.

You can also find listings of board-certified specialists at most public libraries in the *Marquis Who's Who Directory of Medical Specialists* and in the American Board of Medical Specialties (ABMS) directory, the *Compendium of Certified Medical Specialists*. The ABMS also has a toll-free number to call.

In the event that you have any doubts about a doctor, The Public Citizen Health Research Group, run by Sydney Wolff, M.D., based in Washington, D.C., will help you find out if he or she has ever been disciplined by state or federal authorities. The activist organization publishes a list appropriately called *Questionable Doctors*.

Addresses and phone numbers for these sources can be found in Appendix III.

GETTING A COMPREHENSIVE
MEDICAL WORKUP

If you have no risk factors for heart disease, you need only have a complete physical examination and lab workup every few years. If you have any coronary risk factors, it's best to see your doctor at least annually. Some screening tests should be done yearly and are paid for by many HMOs.

During a complete physical, your doctor should take a detailed medical history and conduct a thorough examination, including a number of laboratory tests. Your basic workup should include:

Blood Pressure Check: Once a year for all adults. For people with high blood pressure, diabetes or cardiovascular disease, more frequent monitoring is needed. Blood pressure for a healthy woman should be no higher than 140/90 mmHg.

Serum Cholesterol Test: Total cholesterol and HDL should be measured at least once every five years in all adults over age twenty. An annual lipid profile is needed if a woman is taking birth control pills or is *not* taking replacement hormones after menopause. Total serum cholesterol should be around 200 mg/dl; HDL should be above 45 mg/dl.

Complete Blood Count (CBC): Annually or at your physician's recommendation. The test measures the red blood cell count (hematocrit); lower values may indicate anemia. Some physicians may recommend testing fibrinogen levels.

Urinalysis: Should be done annually. Screens for excess glucose in the urine, which may signal diabetes, and can also detect early kidney disease.

Thyroid/Thyroid-Stimulating Hormone: At a physician's discretion. Thyroid abnormalities may affect heart function and blood pressure; low thyroid levels can raise serum cholesterol.

Electrocardiogram (EKG): A baseline EKG before age forty for women with a strong family history of heart disease or women with major risk factors, such as diabetes. There is no universal recommendation for annual EKGs in women after age forty or fifty.

Note: In addition to the tests above, all women over age eighteen need to have an annual Pap test, and after age forty, women need regular mammograms. It's also advisable for women to have their bone density assessed at menopause and to be screened for uterine and rectal cancer every year after age fifty.

IF YOU HAVE SIGNS
OF HEART DISEASE

If your doctor suspects that you have cardiovascular disease, he or she may refer you for one or more of the following cardiac tests (all of which are explained in Chapter 12):

- Exercise stress test
- Thallium stress test
- Echocardiogram
- Echo-stress test
- MUGA scan
- Angiography

Make sure you get copies of all test results. Use the personal health history section in the back of this book to keep track of tests and to record your family's history, as well as any risk factors you may have.

MAKING IMPORTANT DECISIONS

If tests reveal the presence of cardiovascular disease, you need to find out all you can about your treatment options. In addition to asking questions of your own physician, you can contact the American Heart Association, the National Heart, Lung and Blood Institute and other helpful organizations (addresses and phone numbers can be found in Appendix III).

This investigation is especially important, because many states have *informed-consent laws*, where patients must sign a document stating they have been fully informed about their treatment, before any treatment can begin.

These days, cost can definitely be a factor in care. Health maintenance organizations and other "managed care" medical plans (which will be part of any new national health-care plan) often favor less aggressive (and less expensive) treatment. You need to know exactly what your plan covers; keep careful records.

If you feel uneasy about a treatment recommendation, get another opinion, preferably from someone at a different facility. Be aware that a physician may refer you to another doctor who's likely to agree with his treatment recommendations, notes Dr. Nina Bickell. She suggests getting a second opinion from a physician who does not rely on your specialist for referrals.

Once you and your physician have agreed on a treatment, stick with it, whether it's a low-fat diet, an exercise regimen, or cholesterol-lowering medication. Don't *ever* stop taking medication on your own for any reason. According to the National Council on Patient Information, 30 to 50 percent of all prescribed medications are taken incorrectly. One patient in five never even fills the prescription. One in seven stops taking the medication too soon, and nearly a third of patients neglect to get prescriptions refilled.

Just because you may be feeling better doesn't mean you don't need your medication anymore. Some women fail to inform their doctor of side effects, others can't afford to buy the drugs they need. Many women simply dislike being on long-term medications. If there's a problem, be honest with your physician. Otherwise, he or she cannot help you.

Finally, *put your health first.* Untold numbers of women forgo treatment, or feel that the money or medical attention should go to another family member, says Jane B. Sherwood, R.N., B.S.N., research nurse manager of the MI Onset Study at the New England Deaconess Hospital in Boston.

Some women hate to inconvenience family members with an illness. Sherwood coordinated a study which found that women remained in local hospitals more than two days longer than men before being transferred to larger facilities for more advanced treatment. While physician attitudes toward women's illnesses could have contributed to the delay, Sherwood notes that some of the women in the study said they were reluctant to leave smaller facilities closer to home, because they didn't want to inconvenience their families. Women often told researchers, "My husband won't drive in the city," or "It's too far for my family to come and visit me."

Women in the study didn't complain as often as men about their pain, and family members may have to work with a physician to make sure a woman is getting appropriate care, says Sherwood.

A mild, uncomplicated heart attack that does little damage to the heart muscle does not necessarily need more high-tech care; in such cases, a community hospital can provide adequate care. The more serious the illness, however, the greater the need for advanced treatment. "If your doctor does recommend more advanced treatment or a transfer to a larger facility, think about yourself and what's going to help you get better right away, not what's convenient for your family," advises Sherwood.

Don't become a victim of your *own* unconscious sexual stereotyping —taking better care of others' health than your own. In the end, *you* are the real guardian of your heart's health.

Appendix I
Food Tables

Each food, in the quantity listed, contains the nutritional values enumerated in its category.

FOOD EXCHANGE LISTS FOR WEIGHT LOSS

STARCHES/BREADS

15 gm carbohydrates
 3 gm protein
   trace fat
80 calories

½ cup cooked pasta
⅓ cup rice
¾ cup unsweetened cereals
1½ cups puffed cereal
3 tbsp wheat germ

1 slice bread
½ NY-style bagel (1 ounce)
½ English muffin, bialy
½ burger/frank bun
1 tortilla

MEAT/PROTEIN

 0 gm carbohydrates
 7 gm protein
 3–5 gm fat
50–75 calories

1 ounce skinless poultry or fish
2 ounces shellfish
1 ounce very lean beef, pork, veal or lamb
¼ cup water-packed tuna or salmon
1 ounce uncreamed or smoked herring
2 medium sardines

2 tablespoons grated Parmesan cheese
1 ounce part skim/low-fat cheese
   (under 5 gm fat per ounce)
¼ cup 1% milk-fat cottage cheese

STARCHES/BREADS

½ cup beans/dried peas
⅓ cup cooked lentils
½ cup starchy vegetables (corn, lima beans,
    peas, winter squash)
3 ounces baked potato
½ cup mashed potato
⅓ cup sweet potato/yam

SNACKS

3 cups air-popped popcorn
5 slices melba toast
6 saltines, small crackers
8 animal crackers
3 2½" graham crackers
½ cup low fat, sugar-free pudding or ice cream

MEAT/PROTEIN

½ cup soft tofu
2 teaspoons peanut butter
1 egg
3 egg whites
½ cup egg substitute

VEGETABLES

 5 gm carbohydrates
 2 gm protein
 0 gm fat
25 calories

½ cup cooked, steamed vegetables
    (green beans, broccoli, carrots, cauliflower,
    eggplant, okra, pea pods, peppers, tomatoes)

½ cup tomato or vegetable juice
1 cup raw vegetables
2 tbsp tomato sauce

Free Vegetables:*
cabbage (white or red)
collard greens
celery, cucumbers
lettuce, salad greens
mushrooms
spinach
radishes
onions
zucchini

FRUITS

15 gm carbohydrates
 0 gm protein
   trace fat
60 calories

1 small fresh fruit (apple, pear, peach, orange,
    nectarine)
½ medium large fresh fruit (grapefruit,
    pomegranate, mango)
⅓ cantaloupe (or 1 cup cubes)
⅛ honeydew melon (or 1 cup cubes)
1 cup raspberries or strawberries
12 cherries
15 grapes
½ cup canned fruit in juice (no sugar)

½ cup low-sugar fruit juice (apple, grapefruit,
    orange)
⅓ cup sweeter fruit juices (grape juice,
    cranberry cocktail, prune juice)
2 teaspoons raisins
3 medium prunes

* These vegetables have less than 20 calories per cup and may be eaten in unlimited quantities.

LOW-FAT MILK/YOGURT

12 gm carbohydrates
 8 gm protein
1–2 gm fat
100 calories

1 cup skim milk
1 cup 1%-fat milk
8 ounces plain/nonfat yogurt
8 ounces low-fat, sugar-free
   fruit yogurt

UNLIMITED FOODS/ BEVERAGES

Unsweetened or diet gelatin
Diet, sugar-free drinks
Herbs, spices and other seasonings
Sugar-free candies, gum
Pickles
Mustard
Vinegar, horseradish
Lime, lemon juice
Garlic
Soy sauce, Worcestershire sauce
Hot sauce, flavor extracts
Sugar substitutes
Low-sodium bouillon

FATS

0 gm carbohydrates
0 gm protein
5 gm fat
45 calories

1 teaspoon margarine
1 teaspoon oil
1 teaspoon mayonnaise
2 teaspoons diet margarine
2 teaspoons diet mayonnaise
1 tablespoon cream cheese
1 tablespoon salad dressing

5 large/10 small olives
1 tablespoon cashew nuts
2 walnuts
6 almonds
10 large/20 small peanuts
2 whole pecans

EXCHANGES FOR ALCOHOLIC BEVERAGES

12 ounces beer = 1 starch, 2 fats
12 ounces lite beer = ½ starch, 1 fat
1½ ounces hard liquor = 2 fats
4 ounces dry red/white wine = 2 fats
4 ounces sweet wine = 1 starch, 2 fats
3½ ounces mixed drink = ½ to 1 starch, 2 fats

Note: The above food exchanges were adapted by NYU from *Exchange Lists for Weight Management*, copyright 1986 by the American Diabetes Association and the American Dietetic Association.

Source: NYU Medical Center Health Education Center.

Appendix II
Making Healthful Food Choices

FAT, CHOLESTEROL AND CALORIE CONTENTS
OF COMMON FOODS

FOOD CHOICES	FAT	SATURATED FAT	CHOLESTEROL	CALORIES
Dairy Products	Grams	Grams	Milligrams	
Skim milk (1 cup)	0.4	0.3	4.0	86
1% low-fat milk (1 cup)	2.6	1.6	10.0	102
2% low-fat milk (1 cup)	4.7	2.9	18.0	121
Whole milk (1 cup)	8.2	5.1	33.0	150
Egg, 1 whole	5.6	1.7	274	79
Egg, 1 white	0	0	0	16
Egg Beaters (¼ cup)	0	0	0	25
American cheese (1 ounce)	8.9	5.6	27.0	106
American cheese, "Lite" (1 ounce)	2.5	1.5	10.0	50
American cheese fat-free (1 ounce)	0	0	5.0	45
Swiss cheese (1 ounce)	7.8	5.0	26.0	107
Cheddar cheese (1 ounce)	9.4	6.0	30.0	114
Ricotta, part skim (½ cup)	9.0	5.6	25.0	156
Ricotta, whole milk (½ cup)	14.7	9.4	63.0	216
Cream cheese (1 ounce)	9.9	6.2	31.0	99
Cream cheese, "Lite" (Neufchatel)	6.6	4.2	22.0	74
Mozzarella, nonfat (1 ounce)	0	0	5.0	35

FOOD CHOICES	FAT	SATURATED FAT	CHOLESTEROL	CALORIES
Dairy Products	Grams	Grams	Milligrams	
Mozzarella, part skim (1 ounce)	4.5	2.9	16.0	56
Mozzarella, whole milk (1 ounce)	6.1	3.7	22.0	69
Parmesan, grated (1 ounce)	8.5	5.4	22.0	59
Feta cheese (1 ounce)	6.0	4.2	25.0	75
Cottage cheese, creamed (½ cup)	5.1	3.2	17.0	117
1% low-fat cottage cheese (½ cup)	1.2	0.7	5.0	82
Low-fat yogurt, plain (½ cup)	0.2	0.1	2.0	63
Plain yogurt (½ cup)	3.7	2.4	14.0	70
Frozen yogurt, fruit-flavored	2.0	0.0	0.0	110
Ice cream, soft serve (1 cup)	22.5	13.5	153.0	377
Ice cream, 16% fat (1 cup)	23.7	14.7	88.0	349
Ice milk (1 cup)	5.6	3.5	18.0	184
Cream, heavy (2 tablespoons)	11.0	6.8	42.0	106
Cream, whipped (2 tablespoons)	2.0	1.0	4.0	54
Half and half (2 tablespoons)	4.0	2.2	12.0	40
Sour cream (1 tablespoon)	3.0	1.9	10.0	26
Meats (3½-ounce portion)				
Beef liver, braised	4.9	1.9	389.0	161
Chuck, arm pot roast, lean only	10.0	3.8	101.0	231
Short loin, T-bone or porterhouse steak, lean broiled	10.4	4.2	80.0	214
Brisket, lean only, braised	12.8	4.6	93.0	241
Ground, lean, broiled medium	18.5	7.2	87.0	272
Leg of lamb, lean, roasted	8.2	3.0	89.0	191
Lamb, loin chop, lean, broiled	9.4	4.1	94.0	215
Fresh pork, loin, tenderloin, lean only, roasted	4.8	1.7	93.0	166
Cured, ham, boneless, roasted	9.0	3.1	59.0	178
Fresh, leg (ham), rump, roasted	10.7	3.7	96.0	221
Spare ribs, lean and fat, braised	30.1	11.45	121.0	395
Veal loin chop, lean only	6.7	0.00	90.0	207
Veal cutlet, medium fat, broiled	11.0	4.8	128.0	271

continued

FOOD CHOICES	FAT	SATURATED FAT	CHOLESTEROL	CALORIES
Poultry (3½-ounce portion)	Grams	Grams	Milligrams	
Turkey, roasted, light meat, no skin	1.9	0.4	86.0	140
Turkey, roasted, light meat, w/skin	4.6	1.3	95.0	164
Turkey, roasted, dark meat, no skin	4.3	1.4	112.0	162
Turkey, roasted, dark meat, w/skin	7.1	2.1	117.0	182
Chicken, broilers or fryers, light meat, no skin, roasted	4.5	1.3	85.0	173
Duck, flesh only, roasted	11.2	4.2	89.0	201
Lunch Meats (3½-ounce portion)				
Beef salami, 3 or 4 slices	20.0	10.2	65.0	240
Fresh, Italian sausage, cooked	25.7	9.0	78.0	323
Cured, liver sausage (liverwurst)	28.5	10.6	158.0	326
Cured, smoked link sausage, grilled	31.8	11.3	68.0	389
Cured, salami, dry or hard	33.7	11.9	0.0	407
Bacon, fried	49.2	17.4	85.0	576
Fish and Seafood (3½-ounce portion, cooked)				
Haddock, baked*	0.9	0.2	74.0	112
Halibut, baked	2.9	0.4	41.0	140
Trout, rainbow, baked	4.3	0.8	73.0	151
Swordfish, baked	5.1	1.4	50.0	155
Tuna, bluefin, baked	6.3	1.6	49.0	184
Salmon, sockeye, baked	11.0	1.9	87.0	216
Lobster	0.6	0.1	72.0	98
Shrimp, mixed species, moist heat	1.1	0.3	195.0	99
Clam, mixed species, moist heat	2.0	0.2	67.0	148

* Most other whitefish such as flounder, cod, pollock, perch, etc. have similar values.

Breads/Cereals/Pasta				
Melba toast, 1 plain	tr	0.1	0	0
Pita, ½ large shell	1.0	0.1	0	165
Corn tortilla	1.0	0.1	0	65
Rye, wheat or white bread, 1 slice	1.0	0.3	0	80
Bagel, 1, 3½" diameter	2.0	0.3	0	200
Hot dog or hamburger bun	2.0	0.5	tr	115
Corn muffin, 1, 2½" diameter	5.0	1.5	23.0	145
Croissant, 1, 4½" by 4"	12.0	3.5	13.0	235
Waffle, 1, 7" diameter	13.0	4.0	102.0	245

FOOD CHOICES	FAT	SATURATED FAT	CHOLESTEROL	CALORIES
Breads/Cereals/Pasta	Grams	Grams	Milligrams	
Corn flakes (1 cup)	0.1	tr	0	98
Corn grits, cooked (1 cup)	0.5	tr	0	146
Oatmeal, cooked (1 cup)	2.4	0.4	0	145
"100% Natural cereal" (w/raisins and dates)	20.3	13.7	0	496
Pasta				
Spaghetti/macaroni, cooked (1 cup)	1.0	0.1	0	155
Egg noodles, cooked (1 cup)	2.0	0.5	50.0	155
Snacks, Sweets, etc.				
Pizza, cheese (⅛ of 15" pie)	9.0	4.1	56	290
Quiche lorraine (⅛ of 8" quiche)	48.0	23.2	285	600
Chocolate pudding (½ cup)	4.0	2.4	4.0	150
Hard candy, 1 ounce	0.0	0.0	0	110
Milk chocolate, plain, 1 ounce	9.0	5.4	6.0	145
Vanilla wafers, 5 cookies 1¾" diameter	3.3	0.9	12.0	94
Chocolate brownie, with icing, 1½" × 1¾" × ⅞"	4.0	1.6	14.0	100
Chocolate chip cookies, 4 cookies 2¼" diameter	11.0	3.9	18.0	185
Angel food cake, 1/12 of 10" cake	tr	1.1	0	125
Pound cake, 1/17 of loaf	5.0	3.0	64.0	110
Cream pie, ⅙ of 9" pie	23.0	15.0	8.0	455
Pretzels, stick, 2¼", 10	tr	tr	0	10
Potato chips, 1 ounce	10.1	2.6	0	147

Sources: U.S.D.A. Human Nutrition Information Service; National Cholesterol Education Program.

Appendix III
Where to Get
Information and Help

FOR INFORMATION ON CARDIOVASCULAR DISEASES

THE AMERICAN HEART ASSOCIATION
7320 Greenville Avenue
Dallas, Texas 75231
800-242-8721

The AHA now offers a new information system for the general public (and medical professionals as well) which you can access by calling a toll-free number: (800) AHA-USA-1 (or see above). Callers will be asked to punch in their area code and the first three digits of their telephone number. This automatically routes the call to a person in their nearest AHA office. You may call this number to get information on heart disease, stroke, high blood pressure and local AHA-sponsored events and programs.

Note: One of the newest programs is "Eating for Healthy Tomorrows," a nutrition education program aimed at older African Americans, teaching heart-healthy eating in the context of traditional cooking. The program is jointly sponsored by the AHA and the American Association of Retired Persons. For information, contact your local AHA office.

American Diabetes Association
1660 Duke Street
Alexandria, Virginia 22314
800-232-3472

American Dietetic Association
216 West Jackson Boulevard
Suite 800
Chicago, Illinois 60606
312-899-0040

National Black Women's Health Project
1237 Ralph Abernathy Boulevard, S.W.
Atlanta, Georgia 30310
800-ASK-BWHP
800-275-2947

The National Heart, Lung and Blood
    Institute
National Institutes of Health
P.O. Box 30105
Bethesda, Maryland 20824
301-251-1222

The National Cholesterol Education
    Program Information Center
National Institutes of Health
P.O. Box 30105
Bethesda, Maryland 20824
301-251-1222

The National High Blood Pressure
    Education Program
National Institutes of Health
P.O. Box 30105
Bethesda, Maryland 20824
301-251-1222

National Stroke Association
8480 E. Orchard Road
Englewood, Colorado 80111-5015
303-771-1700

SUPPORT GROUPS

Mended Hearts (AHA-sponsored support
    group for heart patients)
The American Heart Association
7320 Greenville Avenue
Dallas, Texas 75231
214-706-1442

Young Hearts (support group for cardiac
    patients ages twenty–fifty)
P.O. Box 274
Brookfield, Illilnois 60513
708-387-0918

Zipper Clubs (clubs for people who have
    had heart surgery)
1161 Easton Road
Roslyn, Pennsylvania 19001
215-887-6644

The Stroke Connection (AHA-sponsored
    support network for stroke patients;
    publishes two newsletters, *Stroke
    Connection* and *A Stroke of Luck*, for
    aphasia patients)
American Heart Association
7320 Greenville Avenue
Dallas, Texas 75231
800-553-6321

FOR HELP WITH SMOKING CESSATION

American Cancer Society
1599 Clifton Road, N.E.
Atlanta, Georgia 30329
404-320-3333

American Lung Association
Freedom From Smoking Program
1740 Broadway
New York, N.Y. 10019
212-315-8700

American Institute for Preventive
    Medicine
Smokeless Program
30445 Northwestern Blvd.
Farmington Hills, Michigan 48334
800-345-AIPM
(800) 345-2476

Smokenders
1430 East Indian School Road, Suite 102
Phoenix, Arizona, 85014
800-828-4357

FOR INFORMATION ON PHYSICIANS

American Society of Internal Medicine
1101 Vermont Avenue, N.W.
Washington, D.C. 20005
202-835-2746
Provides listings of board-certified
internists.

American Medical Association
515 North State Street
Chicago, Illinois 60610
312-464-5000
You may write to the AMA to request a
physician profile on any of their
members.

The American Board of Medical
    Specialties
1007 Church Street, Suite 404
Evanston, Illinois 60201
708-491-9091
800-776-CERT (Mon.–Fri. 9 A.M.–6 P.M.
    EST)
Operators answering the toll-free line will
tell you whether a particular doctor is
certified by one of the 24 boards who are
members of ABMS. The group also publishes the Compendium of Certified Medical
Specialists, available at most public
libraries.

The Marquis Who's Who Directory of
    Medical Specialists
Reed Reference Publishing Co.
121 Chanlon Road
New Providence, N.J. 07974
A reference book listing medical specialists in every field. Available at most public libraries.

Questionable Doctors
The Public Citizen Health Research
    Group
2000 P Street, N.W.
Washington, D.C. 20036
202-833-3000
Published annually, lists physicians who
have been disciplined by state or federal
government. Available at most public
libraries.

Appendix IV
Additional Reading

Here is a selection of recently published books on heart disease, women and heart disease and health books that feature information for women.

BOOKS ON HEART DISEASE

The Woman's Heart Book: The Complete Guide to Keeping Your Heart Healthy and What to Do If Things Go Wrong by Fredric J. Pashkow, M.D. and Charlotte Libov, Dutton, 1993.

Dr. Pashkow is medical director of Cardiac Rehabilitation at the Cleveland Clinic Foundation. Libov is a medical writer, who herself underwent surgery for a congenital heart defect. Together, they have put together a readable encyclopedia for women not only about cardiovascular diseases, but other disorders of the heart, including congenital disorders, their diagnosis and treatment.

50 Essential Things to Do When the Doctor Says It's Heart Disease by Fredric J. Pashkow, M.D. and Charlotte Libov, Dutton/Plume, 1994.

A companion paperback guide for heart patients to help them take an active role in treatment.

The Black Health Library Guide to Heart Disease and Hypertension by Paul Jones, M.D. with Angela Mitchell, edited by Linda Villarosa, Henry Holt, 1993.

Dr. Jones is chief fellow of cardiovascular medicine at Loyola University Center; Mitchell is a free-lance writer, and Villarosa is a senior editor at *Essence* magazine, specializing in health. This is the first book on heart disease written specifically for

African Americans, and the first in a series of *Black Health Library Guides*. Others in this ground-breaking series include books on stroke, obesity and diabetes.

The Yale University School of Medicine Heart Book edited by Barry L. Zaret, M.D., Marvin Moser, M.D., and Lawrence S. Cohen, M.D., Hearst Books, 1992.

Everything you could ever possibly want to know about the heart and heart disease is detailed in this huge, but reader-friendly, encyclopedia of heart disease and disorders compiled by top cardiologists at Yale. An especially nice touch is its easy-access "book within a book" reference section on disorders and symptoms.

The American Heart Association Family Guide to Stroke Treatment, Recovery, Prevention by Louis R. Caplan, M.D., Mark L. Dyken, M.D., and J. Donald Easton, M.D., Times Books/Random House, 1994.

The authors are all top experts on stroke: Dr. Caplan is a professor of neurology at Tufts University School of Medicine/New England Medical Center in Boston; Dr. Dyken is professor and chairman of the Department of Neurology at the Indiana University Medical Center; Dr. Easton is professor and chairman of the Department of Clinical Neurosciences at Brown University School of Medicine and physician in chief, Department of Neurology, at Rhode Island Hospital. Like other AHA books, this volume is reader-friendly, informative, and up to date.

Women and Heart Disease, What You Can Do to Stop the Number-One Killer of Women by Edward B. Diethrich, M.D. and Carol Cohan, Times Books, 1992.

Dr. Diethrich is the director and chief of cardiovascular surgery at the Arizona Heart Institute and Foundation in Phoenix, a free-standing clinic devoted to cardiology. The authors discuss gender bias in heart disease, offer a test for assessing personal risk, and detail Dr. Diethrich's own program to help women with cardiovascular disease.

Week by Week to a Strong Heart: An Action Plan for Preventing or Treating Heart Disease and Other Circulatory Problems by Marvin Moser, M.D., Rodale Press/St. Martin's Press, 1992.

Dr. Moser is a clinical professor of medicine at the Yale University School of Medicine. This is a year-long, week-by-week plan for reducing the risks of heart disease. Dr. Moser is a no-nonsense cardiologist whose message is that people need not go to extremes about diet or exercise. The book includes material of special interest to women and the elderly.

The Female Heart: The Truth About Women and Coronary Artery Disease by Marianne J. Legato, M.D., and Carol Colman, Simon and Schuster, 1991.

Dr. Legato is a cardiovascular researcher on the faculty of Columbia University College of Physicians and Surgeons and a practicing cardiologist at St. Lukes/Roosevelt Hospital Center in New York. Colman is a medical writer. The book discusses the issue of gender bias, details the biological differences between men and women and looks at women's special risks in diagnosis and treatment, with many case histories included.

Mayo Clinic Heart Book by Michael D. McGoon, M.D., Editor-in-Chief, William Morrow, 1993.

A comprehensive guide to your heart, from the world-renowned Mayo Clinic cardiology department. The book includes a symptoms guide, a detailed reference to more than 120 commonly prescribed heart and circulatory medications, and a special section on women and heart disease.

Heart Disease and High Cholesterol: Beating the Odds by C. Richard Conti, M.D., and Diana Tonnessen, Addison-Wesley, 1992.
    Dr. Conti is chief of cardiology at the University of Florida College of Medicine. This general guide to reducing heart-disease risks emphasizes diet as the primary means of prevention.

A Patient's Guide to Heart Surgery by Carol Cohan, June B. Pimm, and James R. Jude, Harper Collins, 1991.
    A layman's look at all aspects of heart surgery through the recovery period. A good basic source for women who have been referred for surgery and want to know all they can.

Dr. Dean Ornish's Program for Reducing Heart Disease by Dean Ornish, M.D., Random House, 1990.
    Dr. Ornish, director of the Preventive Medicine Research Institute in Sausalito, California, was the author of a landmark study on how a very low-fat diet, exercise and stress management can shrink plaques in coronary arteries. His study found women had better results than men. This book is a how-to guide based on his research.

The Wellness Book: A Comprehensive Guide to Maintaining Health and Treating Stress-Related Illnesses by Herbert Benson, M.D., Eileen M. Stuart, R.N., M.S., and the staff of the Mind/Body Medical Institute of the New England Deaconess Hospital and Harvard Medical School, Carol Publishing Group/Birch Lane Press, 1991.
    Dr. Benson is the author of the classic *Relaxation Response* and the founder and director of the Mind/Body Institute. This book is a comprehensive, how-to guide to reduce stress and manage stress-related illnesses, including heart disease. It features techniques to help with diet, exercise and stress management.

Your Healing Mind by Reed C. Moskowitz, M.D., William Morrow, 1992.
    Dr. Moskowitz is a clinical assistant professor of Psychiatry at New York University School of Medicine, and founder and director of the Stress Disorders Medical Services Program at NYU Medical Center. His book offers suggestions on managing stress-related disorders including heart disease, high blood pressure and high cholesterol. It also deals with issues such as anger and aggression, which women often have trouble coming to terms with.

BOOKS OF SPECIAL INTEREST TO WOMEN

The Complete Book of Menopause: Every Woman's Guide to Good Health by Carol Landau, Ph.D., Michele G. Cyr., M.D., and Anne W. Moulton, M.D., Grosset/Putnam, 1994.
    The authors are cofounders of Women's Health Associates, a hospital-based group

practice at Rhode Island Hospital, Brown University School of Medicine. They discuss every aspect of menopause (including the pros and cons of hormone replacement) in a detailed, informative format.

The New Our Bodies, Ourselves by the Boston Women's Collective, Simon and Schuster/ Touchstone, 1992.
An update of the classic feminist women's health book, with added material on AIDS.

The Good Housekeeping Illustrated Guide to Women's Health, Kathryn A. Cox, M.D., Medical Editor, Hearst Books, 1995.
A comprehensive volume providing practical, up-to-date information on a wide spectrum of women's health issues, from nutrition, exercise, and sexual health to sexual harassment, domestic violence and women's rights in the health care system.

150 Most-Asked Questions About Menopause: What Women Really Want to Know by Ruth S. Jacobowitz, Hearst Books, 1992.
All about menopause in a question-and-answer format. Just about everything you've ever wanted to know, but never thought to ask.

Estrogen: A Complete Guide to Reversing the Effects of Menopause Using Hormone Replacement Therapy by Lila E. Nachtigall, M.D. and Joan Ratner Heilman, Revised and Expanded Edition, Harper Perennial, 1991.
Dr. Nachtigall is a reproductive endocrinologist at NYU's Women's Health Service and associate professor of obstetrics and gynecology at New York University School of Medicine. This is a new edition of her overview of what hormone-replacement therapy can do for postmenopausal women, and a handbook for coping with menopause.

Women's Health Alert by Sidney M. Wolfe, M.D. and the Public Citizen Health Research Group, with Rhoda Donkin Jones, Addison-Wesley, 1991.
Dr. Wolfe is the director of the Public Citizen Health Research Group and regarded as the Ralph Nader of medicine. Subtitled *What Doctors Won't Tell You*, the book looks at the down side of medications, treatments and devices. Worth a read if you are looking for an alternative opinion.

LOW-FAT COOKBOOKS

Here is a selection of heart-healthy cookbooks, featuring those with recipes for low-fat African-American, Oriental, Mediterranean, Jewish and Mexican cuisines.

The American Heart Association Cookbook, 5th Edition: New and Revised edited by Scott M. Grundy, M.D., Ph.D. and Mary Winston, Ed.D., R.D., Times Books, 1992.
Dr. Grundy, director of the Center for Human Nutrition at Texas Southwestern Medical Center in Dallas, is a foremost authority on diet and cardiovascular disease. This is the classic cookbook many physicians recommend for their heart patients. It now contains more than six hundred recipes, each with a complete nutritional breakdown.

Essence Brings You Great Cooking by Jonell Nash, Penguin, 1994.

Nash, food editor for *Essence* magazine, has created a book that not only celebrates African-American (plus Southern and Caribbean) traditional foods, but has found ways to make them more heart-healthy, as well as easy to prepare. She eliminates the lard and heavy use of salt (and salt pork) to devise lighter, simpler recipes for everything from grits and collard greens to Jamaican "jerk" chicken. Each recipe includes a nutritional breakdown.

100% Pleasure: The Low-Fat Cookbook for People Who Love to Eat by Nancy Baggett and Ruth Glick, Rodale Press, 1994.

If you're convinced that low-fat means low taste, this cookbook will quickly change your mind. Baggett and Glick, both authors of other cookbooks, have created easy-to-follow recipes that not only taste good but are also good to your body.

The American Diabetes Association/American Dietetic Association Family Cookbook, Volume IV: The American Tradition, Prentice Hall, 1991.

The latest in a series of family cookbooks by the ADA, this one has a wide selection of American regional recipes from north to south, east to west that are healthy and yummy. Includes official food-exchange lists for people with diabetes.

The Guiltless Gourmet Goes Ethnic: Italian, French, Mexican, Spanish and Cajun Cuisine for the Health-Conscious Cook by Joy Gilliard and Joy Kirkpatrick, R.D., DCI Publishing, 1990.

A paperback cookbook with a plastic ring binding, perfect to prop up on the counter while you whip up one of the authors' delectable-sounding low-fat ethnic dishes.

Mexican Light Cooking: Easy Healthy, Low-Calorie Recipes from Nachos to Tacos by Kathi Long, Perigee Books/Putnam, 1992.

A cookbook that delivers just what it promises. If you love Tex-Mex, but your waistline doesn't, this one's for you. There's even (incredibly) a lower-fat version of guacamole.

The Love Your Heart Mediterranean Cookbook by Carole Kruppa, Surrey/PGW, 1992.

The author of *The Love Your Heart Low Cholesterol Cookbook* has amassed low-fat recipes from Italy, France, Morocco, Spain and Greece that should satisfy the most gourmet cook.

Light and Healthy Mediterranean Cooking by Judith Wills, HP Books, 1992.

Another heart-healthy cookbook for lovers of Italian, Greek and Mideast cuisine.

Low-Cholesterol Cuisine by Anne Lindsay, Quill Books, 1989.

The author provides two hundred recipes ranging from pizza to paella, from Szechuan dishes to southern buttermilk muffins.

Francine Prince's New Jewish Cuisine, 175 Recipes for the Holidays and Every Day: Traditional and Innovative Recipes Reduced in Fats, Sugar, and Calories by Francine Prince, Perigee Books/Putnam, 1992.

Jewish cooking has come a long way from the days when nothing tasted right without a little chicken fat. This book proves you can have your kuchen and eat it, too.

Shuck Beans, Stack Cakes and Honest Fried Chicken: The Heart and Soul of Southern Cooking by Ronni Lundy, Atlantic Monthly Press, 1991.

Sorry, you won't find a recipe for low-fat oil-fried chicken here. But among the 189 recipes, Lundy provides both traditional versions *and* lower-fat alternatives "without the sin." Not technically a low-fat cookbook, but a nice way to discover new ways of down-home cooking.

Oriental Cooking for the Diabetic by Dorothy Revell, R.D., Japan Publications, 1981.

Although oriental cuisine is generally low-fat, some of the ingredients are off-limits to diabetics. This cookbook, though now more than ten years old, should help people with a yen for classic oriental cooking but who have to watch their diets closely.

Yamuna's Table: Healthful Vegetarian Dishes Inspired by the Flavors of India by Yamuna Devi, Dutton, 1992.

If you love the tastes of Indian cooking, here are two hundred recipes for low-fat, easy-to-prepare dishes without meat. Not just for the vegetarians among us.

Cholesterol-Free Cakes and Cookies by Mabel Cavaiani, Henry Holt/Owl, 1992.

For the sweet tooth, one hundred and sixty recipes for all-time favorite desserts minus cholesterol and with less fat and sugar.

Have Your Cake and Eat It, Too by Susan G. Purdy, William Morrow, 1993.

Susan G. Purdy shows how to remove excess saturated fat and cholesterol from favorite desserts without giving up sweet tooth satisfaction, sharing more than 200 recipes low in fat but high in taste and style.

Index